LESBIAN SEX SECRETS

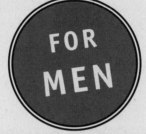

FOR MEN

*What Every Man Wants to Know
About Making Love to a Woman
and Never Asks*

Jamie Goddard
and Kurt Brungardt

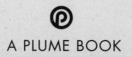

A PLUME BOOK

PLUME
Published by the Penguin Group
Penguin Putnam Inc., 375 Hudson Street,
New York, New York 10014, U.S.A.
Penguin Books Ltd, 27 Wrights Lane,
London W8 5TZ, England
Penguin Books Australia Ltd, Ringwood,
Victoria, Australia
Penguin Books Canada Ltd, 10 Alcorn Avenue,
Toronto, Ontario, Canada M4V 3B2
Penguin Books (N. Z.) Ltd, 182–190 Wairau Road,
Auckland 10, New Zealand

Penguin Books Ltd, Registered Offices:
Harmondsworth, Middlesex, England

First published by Plume,
a member of Penguin Putnam Inc.

First Printing, May, 2000
1   3   5   7   9   10   8   6   4   2

℗ REGISTERED TRADEMARK—MARCA REGISTRADA

LIBRARY OF CONGRESS CATALOGING-IN-PUBLICATION DATA
Goddard, Jamie.
Lesbian sex secrets for men : what every man wants to know about making love to
a woman and never asks / Jamie Goddard and Kurt Brungardt.
p.   cm.
ISBN 0-452-28133-4
1. Sex instruction for men. 2. Women—Sexual behavior. 3. Lesbians—Sexual
behavior. I. Brungardt, Kurt. II. Title.
HQ36.G68616 2000
613.9'6—dc21   99-053311

Printed in the United States of America
Set in Garamond Light

"This book is about how to pleasure women. We all want to know how we can be better lovers of women. Lesbians bring a different and very important perspective to men. These women not only have experience making love to women, but they also live inside female bodies. They know it from the inside out.

"We've all heard the common question, 'So what do lesbians do in bed? Do they really have sex?'

"This book gives you the inside scoop and straight-up advice on pleasing a woman sexually, emotionally, and intimately."

**Be the Best Lover She Has Ever Had
with . . .**

Lesbian Sex Secrets for Men

Jamie Goddard is a sexuality educator, artist, and activist who received her master's degree from New York University in Human Sexuality and Health Education.

Kurt Brungardt is a performance artist and a writer who specializes in health, fitness, and men's issues. He has been featured in *Details*, *Newsweek*, and *The New York Times*, and has appeared on the *Today* show and *20/20*.

For all of my lovers, past, present and future.
You are each a unique inspiration.
—J.G.

For my Aunt Judy who opened new ways of seeing things
and to my future lovers.
—K.B.

CONTENTS

ACKNOWLEDGMENTS

It's amazing how much it takes to create a lil' ol' book. There is no way we possibly could have finessed this one without the support and input of many amazing beings. Neither this book, nor any amount of sanity would have been possible without our unofficial editor and feedback goddess extraordinaire, Jillian Gonzales. From the depths of our spirits, we thank you for your dedication and many hours spent helping us fine-tune this puppy. In the final hours, many illustrious folks gave us the gifts of their sharp minds, insight, and fast typing, as well as true support throughout the process. Shauna, Brian, Ben, Tracy, and Elmar, we appreciate all your hard work.

Huge lumps of gratitude go out to each and every individual who participated in our focus groups or took the time and thought to fill out our surveys. You are too numerous to mention by name, but we thank you all for enriching the book with your voices and experiences, and helping to guide the direction and focus of our writing.

Special thanks also go out to Kimberly Perdue, for bringing fresh energy, many helpful insights, and enthusiasm to the process; to our agent, Dan Strone, for his confidence and guidance; and to Chantal for all her help streamlining the project.

Janene Sneider, we never could've imagined the possibility of such goodness and recollaboration, without your insight and lovely little mirror to reflect our shadows. Thanks for serious realignment and all your advice on the manuscript. Our blessings to you in your own work, soon to be presented to the world.

Aunt Judy and Margaret, thanks for the hospitality and giving us the space to get started.

To everyone at CHP: we graciously appreciate your patience, support and generosity. CHP was an invaluable resource in the materialization of *LSS*. Michael, Jane, Claudia, Jen, Rose, Elliot, Kendra and Ian—you all rock in the advancement of sexuality education. Keep on keepin' on.

Jamie would like to personally thank Shauna and Jillian— your ears, grace, patience, and friendship have been the greatest blessings. Betty Dodson, your mentoring and guidance have helped me dance through this maze and for that I am so grateful . . . from the bottom of my clit, I salute you. Janene, words can't even express how important your insight, guidance, and support are to me. You keep me grounded in reality. Andy, thank you for providing the soundtrack to my writing through the music you have shared with me. WFMU, little do you know how helpful you've been, especially a little Tuesday pioneer named Trouble. Pooka, you have been my queen. Thanks for being my devoted and patient companion. And to Lydia, I don't know if I ever could have taken on such a project without you in my life as teacher, lover, and friend. Thanks for sending me off to do good with what I'd learned. Your presence in this book is immense. Thank you, courageous spirit.

Kurt would like to say thanks to Karen for patiently reading over chapters, editing, and sharing your ideas. Your support and knowledge was invaluable. Michelle, thanks for your humor and input, and sharing your secrets when it comes to . . . you know. Tracy, for being there at crunch time, making unturkey sandwiches, and lending an ear throughout the process. Doug, for a constant well of good advice . . . you are the only person I know who is always right. To DJ, Sammy, and Harold for the boat rides, and for all the meals you cooked, especially those beans, homemade salad dressing, and the egg whites for protein. And to Zoe, thanks for all the walks and ball playing that kept my head clear.

And to all our other friends and family members, who through their love helped propel us in the creation of this book, you are in our hearts and we thank you.

PREFACE

This book brings two traditionally distanced groups to the table to talk about topics they are both interested in and passionate about: women and sex. That was the irony. Kurt wanted to write the book, but not much of a lesbian himself, he needed to find one to help him. He found Jamie, a queer-identified sexuality educator, who agreed that the project sounded like a good idea. We knew that together we could gather a lot of good information and have some fun doing it.

We didn't want to do it alone. We sent out surveys to folks (including heterosexual women), and the responses were fascinating and invaluable. We organized focus groups between heterosexual men and lesbian/bisexual women. The lesbians and the men had a lot to talk about and those conversations informed our writing. Some groups went smoothly as the men and women related to each other with the utmost respect and genuine interest; others were rocky and stressful as the chasms between heterosexual men and lesbian/bisexual women became clear. The voices of heterosexual women are included because it was important to hear their desires and frustrations about sex. People shared a lot of personal stuff with us, and for that we thank you all.

We wrote this book as a queer woman and heterosexual man who have vested interests in helping men love women better. The book is from our combined perspectives and does not speak for all lesbians, nor for all men. Both worlds are far too complex to capture in a subjective book like this. We are two people, each with our own lens on the world. The other voices enhance the book, but ultimately it comes from us. This book is a primer, to help people begin thinking and talking about sex in a new way.

You will find variety in the language we use. We will call genitals "vulvas" and "penises" on one page, "pussies" and "cocks" on the next. We understand that not everybody is comfortable with all these terms. Some people never name their genitals, but it's important to name our parts! How else can we be specific enough to get our needs met? How can you and your lover talk about what you like if you always call it "down there"? "Honey, I love it when you touch me down there, but I don't like it when you run your digits over my backside." The language you choose to use or not use can be a hindrance. We use the words because we like them, and we hope that by using them we desensitize them a bit, so they won't be so threatening for some.

Pay special attention to our "Honey, Come Closer" tips. They are an invitation to lean in so we can share with you crucial and juicy pieces of information about sex with women. It is our mission to help people find more bliss and depth in the energetic exchange of sex. We chose to do that by connecting two groups of people who do not always connect or understand each other. There is not enough dialogue between straight men and gay women. That in itself made this project worth doing. If sex can open up that dialogue, then maybe from there we can create some sensitivity for our different experiences, a deeper understanding, and higher level of respect for each other.

One thing we can all agree on is that women are complex creatures. We love them, but they drive us nuts. We want them, but they don't always want us. We get one, and we don't know what to do with her. This book is a guide to how you can nurture, heal, love, and fuck your female partner to the satisfaction of both of you. So sit back and enjoy!

Jamie and Kurt, September 1999

The Lesbian
Classroom

Introduction

This book is about how to pleasure women. We think lesbians and heterosexual men have a lot in common right there—we all want to know how we can be better lovers of women. Lesbians bring an important perspective to men: They not only have experience making love to women, but they also live inside female bodies. They know it from the inside out.

There are fundamental advantages to this perspective. Research has shown that lesbians have orgasms more often in partner sex than heterosexual women. Okay, men, time to step up to the plate! Most of the women who participated in our focus groups did so because they sincerely want to help men be better lovers of women. Many lesbians have been on the other side and know that a lot of men could use a helping hand.

The women came to the groups not to divulge secrets, but to share tips and express what they've learned about making love to women. This kind of exchange is rare, and some of the ideas may be new, but they aren't really *secrets* per se. Otherwise they wouldn't be shared! What we found was that the real secret to being able to pleasure women is to have the space for open, courageous communication about sex.

What's a Lesbian?

Okay, first things first: What's a lesbian? This is actually a more complicated question than it seems. All women who love women do not fall into one neat little category. There is a wide range of experience and identities within the tribe. You can't necessarily pick them out on the street. You've probably talked to

> ### ♡ Honey, Come Closer
>
> Honey, there's fantasy and there's reality. The reality is that no magic potion, button, tongue swirl, strap-on, or vibrating toy takes the place of you as an attentive and caring lover. There are no shortcuts. The best way to keep any woman interested in you is to be genuinely interested in her and her pleasure!

one before without knowing she was a lady-lover. There might be one in your family. Maybe you're one of those guys who fell in love with one.

There are many variations on sexual orientation for women. Some women call themselves "lesbian"; some prefer "bisexual," "pansexual," "sexual," "queer," "gay" or simply identify themselves as lovers of women, refusing any of these labels. For ease, we will refer to all of these women as "lesbians." All of the women have had sex with other women, which we will refer to as "lesbian sex." Sexual orientation just isn't as simple as box A, B, or C anymore.

The Lesbian World: Fantasy and Reality

Why are lesbians so fascinating? In part, because most people's idea of what lesbians are is skewed. But there's also something pretty damn hot about women loving and sucking on other women. You, like most heterosexual men, find something about lesbians provocative enough that you picked up this book, and chances are, you've entertained your own version of the woman-woman fantasy. Even Howard Stern named the first chapter in his first book after lesbians, as well he should, since he spends so much airtime talking about them! He says, "Lesbianism, let's face it, is a godsend. Every man in the world is totally fascinated by those sisters of Sappho. I know I am." Well, maybe not every man in the world, but probably most of the men who will read this book.

But Howard follows this statement with the typical male reason for digging lesbians: "To have two girls doing wild things to each other with me in the sack would be unbelievable." In the fantasy, the guy always gets to be involved in lesbian sex, but this is a far cry from reality. When two women have sex, they want to be with each other! Many men will assume women need a penis to consummate the experience. They've been watching too much bad porn. Yet that is the very thing that many men find so fascinating about lesbian sex: If there's no penis, it must be different, right?

Learning to Sex It Up

We've all heard the question "So what *do* lesbians do in bed? Do they *really* have sex?" Honey, please. If you've fallen into the all-too-common trap of thinking that sex equals a penis-in-a-vagina, read on. Without the standard heterosexual roles, lesbians have a wide-open road to create whatever roles and whatever kinds of sex they want. That is a big part of why lesbian sex is so hot.

Sex is learned. Our values and beliefs about sex, how we perform sex and experience our sexuality, are all learned behaviors and ideas. We don't come into the world thinking women should achieve orgasm through vaginal penetration, that anal sex is disgusting, that oral sex is the ultimate, that big dicks are better, that abortion is wrong, that lesbians are really hot or really gross, that our bodies are desirable or not. We get messages from our cultures that tell us these things, feed our ideas about sexuality, and teach us what is acceptable and unacceptable behavior.

Lesbians learn about sex differently from heterosexual men or women because of the wider range of roles, because of homophobia, and because it's just a different ball o' wax. While growing up some lesbians learn that being lesbian is wrong or sinful, while others learn to celebrate their sexuality from the get-go. These early messages will clearly have a big impact on how a lesbian experiences her love for women as she gets older. At the same time, some bisexual women learn that they must choose between heterosexuality and gayness, that they are traitors (to both communities), or that they have the best of all worlds and are allowed to choose partners as they wish with no guilt. Each lesbian or bisexual woman will have her own twist, since all lesbians do not learn in the same way any more than all heterosexual men, women, gay men, Muslims, or kids who grow up in Ohio do.

The Lesbian Intervention

There are many things about sex and relationships that my partners, friends, and family just didn't or couldn't teach me. In some cases, what they did teach was more damaging than helpful.　　　　　—Doug, 28, Baltimore

Okay, there is a lot of confusion out there. Men and women need an outside group to help them build a bridge—to jump-start that frank dialogue. Lesbians are in a unique and somewhat objective position to teach men about pleasing a woman sexually, emotionally, and intimately. Not only are lesbians outside the quagmire of the heterosexual battleground; they have neither the desire nor the need to pander to and humor men. So they can give straight-up advice.

I learned more about sex from my first lesbian lover than I did from any of my other partners. Seems like there's plenty to learn from lesbians for both men and women.
　　　　　—Fina, 52, Charlottesville, Virginia

We know there is much you can learn from women's intimate approaches to other women. Obviously you think so too, or you wouldn't have picked up this book. If it was a gift and you're reading it out of obligation or with skepticism, that's good. Keep reading—we promise you'll learn *something*.

One heterosexual woman who received our survey wrote back, totally horrified by the whole idea: "What do lesbians think they can teach men about how to have sex with women?" The question is more aptly put: What *can't* lesbians teach men about sex with women? The implication is that lesbians don't have penises, so how can they teach men to fuck?

Well, that's a common misconception and a perfect illustration of what this book is about. Or isn't about. This book, as crazy as the whole idea may seem, won't be focusing on penises. At least, it will talk about the penis in a whole new way, and you might actually find it refreshing.

One guy wrote to share the story of his sexual initiation. We felt it was so poignant and knew that many men would relate to it. If you still aren't sure why we wrote this book, the following story may help explain.

> *When I think about how I felt about sex when I was growing up, I remember never knowing what it really was about. I knew what it was, but I had no idea how to do it. I had friends who talked about it all the time, and I remember lying and saying that I had done it too. The first time I had the chance to do it was when I was sixteen. She was a virgin at that time too. I was so worked up about the whole thing that when we were finally going to have sex, I couldn't even get it up. She wasn't worried about it, but at the time I thought I looked like the biggest idiot. She just wanted to be with me.*
>
> *I never called her or talked to her again after that day until I was 20. She called lots of times and even wanted me to go to her prom. I put up a wall around me because of that incident. I was so afraid to get naked with a girl after that, and it destroyed my self-esteem. I thought that there was something wrong with me. I even went to a doctor to find out if there was. It just turned out that I was so worried about impressing this girl with some big dick like all the stories I'd heard from so many friends that I couldn't do it.*
>
> *I had no conception that a girl could like me for who I am. I thought I had to be some tough guy who knew how to use his tool. If I had had someone to tell me how to have sex and even given me condoms to use, that would have changed my life.* —Bryan, 23, Pensacola, Florida

Had this young man known that, with or without a hard-on, he could please his lover in myriad ways so that both of them could walk away gleefully satisfied, his sexual learning would have been altered dramatically. Had someone explained that if he hung in there and tried other activities, focusing on his partner for a while, exploring her body and not worrying about his dick, he probably would have gotten a rise from the great turn-on of her arousal. If someone had told him what great sexual tools his brain, mouth, and hands are, he might have been a changed youth. But most of us don't get taught about sex like that. In fact, most men walk around for years and sometimes their whole lives with the social and cultural pressure to know exactly what to do when they "get in a girl's pants" and to be a big-dicked dynamo when it happens. But how can you know if you've never been taught?

This book focuses on lesbian and bisexual women who celebrate, embrace, and want to share their sexuality. They are sharing with you great gifts of their culture. Accept the gift, sit back, and read to your body and mind's content. Allow it to take your learned ideas and sex practices to another place and give you a new way of looking at sexuality, women, and your own sexual person. We hope the book is helpful. It is a privilege for you to get to peer into the sexual lives of this group of women, and when you are finished, maybe you'll appreciate lesbians in a whole new way.

Welcome to the lesbian classroom. Open your mind, pay attention, and take detailed notes. Get ready to be broken down and built back up with love and an occasional kick in the pants. You're going to learn a lot more than how to go down on a woman. You're also going to learn to communicate and see the female body in a refreshing new way. If you improve the way you think about sex, you change the way you perform it. You're going to be a better man for it!

Okay, let's get to it.

First Things First: The Whole Woman

☀ More Than Lip Service

For me, when communication isn't happening, the situation becomes very dissatisfying. If I don't know what she wants (or he, when I've been sexual with men), or vice versa, we end up trying to second-guess each other and it isn't as gratifying as it could be. —Rena, 41, Toronto

Lesbians are well known for their processing. The Sapphic sisters tend to discuss and emotionally process everything, from when to merge bank accounts and rent a U-Haul, to the cultural effects of the latest socially conscious film, to how they felt about last night's romp. They talk. Talk, talk, talk, talk, talk. Sometimes to a fault, overprocessing and running clarity into the ground. That's how the stereotype goes, anyway. It's certainly true to a great extent. But remember, the thing about stereotypes is that they "typify" people, and there are always exceptions. If women tend to be more verbal in general, then two women together is going to mean more discussing, communicating, and mouth-to-mouth action. Lesbians know about more than one kind of oral sex! It's a good thing, because many people don't talk—not *really*.

♡ Honey, Come Closer

Your most important sex organ isn't between your legs. It's between your ears.

Communication, ooh la la . . . it's the reason you bought the book, right? If you are ready to skip to the juicy stuff, stop! If you have an aversion to this section for any reason, then that's the very reason you must read it. And if you are a man who is excited about learning to communicate about sex better, then serious kudos to you. Needless to say, communication is the number one way to find out what your partner likes. Its importance can't be overstressed. One thing is for sure: Communication is not easy for most people. It takes practice and work to get good at it. This is one area where lesbians can definitely share the knowledge.

> *When there are issues between lovers and communication is shut down, sex suffers. How often was it that the first place you realized there was trouble in your relationship was in bed, when your partner was not really responding? Communication about sex is a complex business; there are layers and levels of meaning, and in the end it should be an onion-peeling process: I reveal a layer for you, you reveal a layer for me. Where there is trust combined with curiosity and healthy libidos, spontaneous combustion is sure to follow.*   —Lee, 54, Northbrook, Illinois

Nobody said it was easy. Far from it. Talking about what is right and wrong in a relationship, especially when it comes to sex, is sticky business. Even just talking about what we like or want can be hard, because we don't always learn to ask for what we want. Many emotions—like embarrassment or guilt—can come into play, adding more pressure. But once you break the ice, the ride gets a whole lot easier.

Language: Good Words, Bad Words?

> *I don't know how to talk about sex. I feel crude when I say "cunt," "pussy," "tits," "cock." And I feel nerdy and clinical when I say "vagina," "clitoris," "breasts," "penis."*
> —Dan, 28, Atlanta

Anytime I talk about a woman's appearance I feel like a pig. To physicalize a woman in any way makes me feel evil. So how am I supposed to talk about sex? I don't feel like I have the right to talk about a woman, at least not in front of a woman, like she might pull rank or something. So I've just shut up.   —Jim, 23, San Francisco

It's hard to talk about sex, really hard. The language is so charged. Sexual language can shame us, make us feel guilty and dirty. It can also excite us and help us get in touch with our sexuality and our bodies. Our society is plagued with a conflicted attitude toward sex and the body. Most sex words are considered "dirty words," or they carry negative connotations. Sex words, especially those associated with our bodies and sexual acts, are *normally* used as insults. So it's time to be *abnormal* and use them in a positive way. There is a strange irony in our using as insults words that give us so much pleasure.

When someone is weak or wimpy, they're called a "pussy." When someone is being totally obnoxious, they're called a "dick" or an "asshole." Anger is often expressed with phrases like "fuck you" or "cocksucker." And one common insult is "Suck my dick." Because this language is so negatively charged, it's hard to participate in the acts they describe with pure joy and pride. Even if we feel we are beyond this, the negative overtones reverberate at the unconscious level. So we need to make an effort to clean out our unconscious closet.

The first step in sexual communication is purging the words of their negative qualities and endowing them with positive feelings, taking back the language of sex and owning it as many gay folks have done with the words "queer," "dyke," or "fag." Of course, the words carry a very different meaning when outsiders use them. We need to take the language back and see it as a positive source of communication, and not as a way to create shame and hurl insults. When you first start to talk about sex, using this provocative language may make you feel awkward and shy; but with repetition and a good attitude, the joy, eroticism, and power inherent in the words will come shining through.

You will find that many of your female partners won't even know what to call their own genitals. Many women haven't found words they are comfortable with yet, and that's often because they are not comfortable with their genitals, period. You may have to work with each sexual partner you have to find words that work for both of you.

:♡: Honey, Come Closer

Each time you're with a new lover you have to create a new language. You have to find a way to talk about love and sex that opens you up and excites you both.

Why do we have to talk about it?

While we were having sex I was, for the first time, vocal about what I wanted her to do—namely, to be inside me. I feel like a different person now that I have had sex in something other than silence.   —Michelle, 30, New York

Sharing fantasies after sex is a great way to learn about each other when you feel the closest and most open.
                                                    —Ali, 27, Tucson

Now, if you are one of those people who think talking about sex ruins the mood, destroys the moment, is an interruption, or is not sexy, throw those ideas out the window! Truly. Talking about sex before you ever get naked with someone can be the hottest prelude, the best foreplay, and pretty good insurance that you'll have a mutually satisfying experience. It doesn't mean it will be perfect, but sharing with your partner your likes and dislikes, what you want to try, and where your boundaries are will give you both a lot more to work with than fumbling hands, silence, and lack of mental connection.

Just about 100 percent of the people we've spoken with while writing this book have sworn by this. The other thing that

> ### ☼♡☼ Honey, Come Closer
>
> The one thing that is as clear as the windows after spring cleaning is that *communication is the key to good sex!* You've got to learn how to do it to be a great lover.

became clear is that folks need to do a lot of work on communicating about sex. Not just men, women too, although the consensus seems to be that men need a little extra push. One woman put it frankly: "Men suck at communication." Now, we know that there are men out there who are amazing communicators, so keep up the good work—this will be a refresher for you. For those who need some work in this area, let's get down to business.

Communication Tips

How do you actually go about talking about sex? Especially if you've never done it? For starters, be honest with your partner. Tell her it's hard for you to talk about sex, but it's important to you and you want to try. Just break the ice. Once you do, it will be hard to go back. If you start a relationship with open and sensitive communication, chances are you will continue with the good habits throughout. It's much harder to start out not communicating and then try to incorporate it later. Set the tone right away when you start something new.

> *I think it would be good if men could feel secure enough about themselves to actually ask about how I'm enjoying what they're doing, what I would prefer, what I like, etc. I think this type of dialogue opens people up to potential negative criticism—which people definitely don't want in the bed—so they are not likely to open the communication channel at all.*   —Marissa, 30, Chino Hills, California

I just tell the truth and am very detailed. I tell my partner exactly what I like, what bothers me, and how WE can make it better. It's important to say how WE can fix a problem, especially a sex problem. It takes the pressure off.
　　　　　　　　　　　　　—Lissette, 24, New York

By opening up a dialogue with your partner about how to please her sexually, not only are you becoming a better-attuned lover by the minute; you are also showing her that you care about her pleasure, and that is what most women want.

When talking sex, keep the following guidelines in mind:

- *Use a gentle approach.* Most people feel pretty vulnerable when discussing such delicate and personal matters.
- *Encourage your lover to tell you what she likes.* Many people, especially women, are not used to expressing what they want or like sexually and need help to overcome their shyness.
- *Don't discuss sexual problems or issues during or right after sex.* It's always best to discuss them in a nonsexual context, such as over a meal, so they are less threatening and you both are not as vulnerable.
- *Choose an appropriate time to bring up issues.* Do it when you will both have time to have a full discussion. If she has to be somewhere in 45 minutes, then hold off. It's not fair to start something important knowing you won't be able to finish.
- *Approach the conversation with the intent to find a solution.* If you keep that goal in mind at every turn, you will keep your attitude in check and avoid going the negative, finger-pointing route.
- *Actively listen.* It's not as easy as it sounds. Active listening means responding without interrupting, making eye contact, reflecting what you are hearing and not thinking about what you are going to say next while she is talking. Take a step back and listen to what she is saying to you. It's important. You would want her to do the same. Re-

member, there is a reason we have two ears and one mouth!

- *Use "I" statements:* "I feel frustrated when you shut down and won't tell me what you like." "My needs are not getting met, and I'd like to discuss this with you." You take responsibility for your feelings and actions when you use "I" statements.
- *Avoid placing blame.* Instead of saying "You make me angry, and that's why I flip out on you," try this approach: "I feel angry when you shut down and won't have sex with me and won't talk to me about it. Would you please talk to me about what's going on so we can resolve this situation?" Make an "I" statement; then make a request for what you need from her.
- *Do not use put-downs:* "You've never given me a good blow job." Especially when talking about sexuality, put-downs are really damaging to your partner and may affect her level of trust in the relationship.
- *Avoid making comparisons to other lovers:* "My last girlfriend gave me better head than you ever have."
- *Reflect back to her what you hear her saying.* Sometimes what somebody says and what the other person hears are not the same thing. You can avoid misunderstandings by clarifying what she says: "So what I'm hearing you say is that it upsets you that the only time I want to have sex with you is when I am intoxicated." Then she can let you know if that's what she really meant, or she can rephrase it so it is clearer. Reflection can alleviate 95 percent of miscommunication between people if both parties actively listen and reflect back to each other what they hear.
- *Follow up.* After you've discussed sexual issues and had time to process the talk and put it into practice, check in to see how she's feeling about it now that some time has passed, what improvements have been made, and what still might be lacking or needs further discussion or attention. Don't make the mistake of waiting too long to follow up.

- *Understand that outside forces can affect your sex life.*
  Both of you bring personal issues into the bedroom that
  can affect what goes on in there. For instance, if your lover
  is uncomfortable with her body, she might be self-conscious
  during sex and may even avoid certain acts or sexual situations because of it. This has nothing to do with you, but
  it may seem like it does, and you might have a hard time
  not taking it personally. Try to see what the *real* roots of
  problems are.

Listening

Men, you have no small task ahead. Even the most "sensitive
guys" often talk way too much. Then many women complain
that you clam up when they really want to understand where
you are coming from and that you don't express your feelings at
all. Put some effort into learning to listen—to yourself, to your
body, to your partner, to her body, to the dynamic between you
and the sexual energy you create. You are truly powerful when
you can do that.

> *Communication with your lover . . . getting to know what
> someone is about, creating vulnerability when we talk
> about sexual satisfaction . . . no vulnerability . . . no real
> satisfaction. It's the difference between mutual masturba-
> tion and the intensity of intimacy. . . . It all begins with
> asking questions and getting answers . . . It can start inno-
> cently, when did you get your first kiss . . . realize you
> wanted to touch your first . . . felt like you wanted to break
> the rules and . . . your lover will feel seen and that you are
> actually making love to her.*   —Janene, 50, New York

Does it sound simple? It is. But it's not easy. Learning to tune
in and listen, inquire and wait for the answers, is the most crucial key to satisfying sex and relationships. Period. There are a
lot of women who need to learn to listen and tune in too, but
on the whole, women are the ones who have been silenced, or

have silenced themselves and have had to go inward—listening, nurturing, tuning in internally, and being a wide-armed vessel for the emotions of those they love. Talking is a two-way street.

Discussing Safer Sex

I'd never have sex without talking about it first. It's difficult to always initiate the negotiations, but easy to state my wants and boundaries. If that's not easy to do, I don't know that I want to be having sex with that person.
      —Julia, 22, Westchester County, New York

Safer sex is not an easy topic to bring up for many people, but it's crucial that you do bring it up. There is so much anxiety for people when presented with a prospective new lover. "Will he use a condom?" "Will she expect me to have condoms?" "What will she say if I ask her to use protection for oral sex?" "I'm afraid of getting an STI [sexually transmitted infection]—how do I know she's safe?" "I don't want to get pregnant, but we haven't discussed birth control."

All this anxiety does not make sex more enjoyable. If you and your partner are preoccupied with worries about safety and risk, it will detract from the pleasure of the experience, since your head will be somewhere else and you won't be able to be fully present. As difficult as it may be to bring up safer sex before having sex with a partner, it will have many positive effects. It will get you off on a positive foot by opening the lines of communication from the start, and that will begin to build trust. Whatever the duration or arrangement of the relationship, it will be much richer if you are communicating. Generally, people continue in patterns that start early in a relationship, and sometimes they can be hard to change once they are set. So if you begin communicating openly about expectations, safety, and history, it will be much easier to continue to have open dialogue about these important topics.

When broaching the subject of safer sex, it's best to first have a clear idea of what is and is not acceptable for you. If you're clear on your boundaries, you will be able to express them and have them respected. So if you haven't had that discussion with yourself yet, have it.

Things to discuss with your partner

- *When to use protective barriers (condoms, gloves, dental dams, etc.).* All the time, or for certain sex acts? What risks are you not willing to take?
- *The method of birth control you will use and any special needs around its use.* Men do not often get involved with issues around birth control other than bringing the condoms. Condoms are the only method that will protect from unwanted pregnancy *and* sexually transmitted infections (STIs). If she also uses another contraceptive method, ask her about it and make it your responsibility too. It's important for men to be involved in reproductive-health issues.
- *HIV status and the last time each of you was tested.* You want to discuss when your last unprotected sexual act occurred, if at all. If you had unprotected (without a latex or other barrier) oral, anal, or vaginal sex and have not been tested for HIV, you could be at risk, and it is your partner's right to know this information so she can decide what she needs to do for her own safety. She should share the same information with you.
- *Sexual history, including most recent partners, what risks you have put yourselves at, and whether you've ever had an STI.* Be honest about your history. This doesn't mean you have to tell her everything you've ever done, but you should share the important stuff with her, and she should share with you. Your sexual lives did not begin when you met each other. We all have a past. Own it and be honest about it.
- *If either of you has an STI (e.g., herpes, HPV, HIV):* What behaviors are you willing to engage in and how will you protect yourselves? It can be hard to admit to having an STI because there is so much stigma attached. Having an

STI doesn't mean you're irresponsible. Things happen. You are irresponsible only if you have one and don't share that information with your partner and therefore put her at risk or don't respect her boundaries.

- *Whether you currently have other sex partners and what risks you take with them.* Again, come clean. This doesn't mean you have to share intimate details about your sexual relationships with other partners, but everyone should be on the same page about what's happening and any risks involved.
- *Your expectations of each other.* Be clear about what you want from each other, your boundaries and what level of respect you expect.

Safer sex may be a hard subject to bring up, but don't let your fears or awkwardness prevent you from talking it out. Both of you will probably find yourselves incredibly relieved. It will be worth it in the long run to protect yourself and your partners. And it can be hot foreplay to discuss details of what sexual acts you'd like to engage in safely. You will learn a lot about your partner from this conversation, and the sex will be that much more pleasurable. You'll both be clear about boundaries and what you each want to get out of it, and you won't be spending time worrying about whether you are going to contract something or have an unintended pregnancy. Instead, you'll be able to focus on each other's body and pleasure.

☼♡☼ *Activity:* Gauging Desire

You and your partner can do a simple activity to get on the same page. Think of it as a helpful sexual get-to-know-you. All you need is paper and a writing utensil. Finish the following statements independently and then come together and share your answers.

1. Sexually, the things I like or would like to try are . . .
2. Sexually, the things I do not like and am not interested in doing are . . .
3. Sexually, the gray areas I am unsure of, but would like to explore, are . . .

Sharing and comparing what you wrote will allow you to have an honest discussion about boundaries, so you can be clear about what you each do and do not like and what areas you can begin to explore together. By discussing these three simple things, you will have a whole arsenal of information with which to proceed in your sexual relationship. This is also a helpful exercise for anyone interested in beginning to explore any aspects of S/M, which we'll discuss later in the book.

☀ Opening Up

I think I am afraid to be open about my feelings, for fear of ridicule or misunderstanding, or fear of hurting my partner's feelings. —Judy, 20, Stamford, Connecticut

I think women (at least most of them) take sex to a more mental place than men. It means more, connecting to each other. —Chriss, 31, New York

♡ Honey, Come Closer

If you want to learn to pleasure a woman, connect to her in more ways than one, as a whole person. You have to open up and let her in.

Trust

The first step is establishing trust with someone. You can't
have good sex if you don't trust that person.
> —Tonya, 26, Bryan, Texas

To discuss opening up emotionally we must discuss the notion of trust. Our ability to let go emotionally is linked to how
much we trust ourselves and the people we are with. How can
a woman let go if she doesn't feel emotionally, psychologically,
and physically safe? Trust is a necessary component for safety.

Creating trust starts by building a connection verbally. This
again is where lesbians come out ahead, because although they
may process things to death, that processing requires a high
level of communication, which builds trust, and lovers begin to
see more dimensions of each other, feel safe enough to let go,
and experience more pleasure.

The best sex I ever had was with my best friend, and what I
think made the sex so great was not only his ability to per-
form, but also the level of trust we had achieved with one
another because we were best friends. I could do all sorts of
things with him I wouldn't have necessarily done with any-
one else because I knew that after we had our round of
great sex or what-not, he wouldn't leave me, and he would
still be there emotionally for me. I think trust is really a part
of great sex.   —Violarium, 18, Clemson, South Carolina

If there is honest communication, trust is being built. If a
woman trusts, she can really let go. In letting go, she releases
whatever may hinder her and can be totally present with you.
With presence and release, she becomes open to powerful orgasms. If you have a lover who is unable to reach orgasm, that
may be linked to how much or how little trust and connection
you have. This is not always the case. Sometimes orgasm is
strictly physical, and it works just fine. Other times it requires a
higher level of interaction and understanding with a lover. But

ultimately, for there to be real trust, talk has to be backed up by action. Walk your talk!

> *Physical sex can still be great, but physical/emotional sex is even more intense, since each of you is more interested in how to please your partner. I also think that when you're emotionally involved with someone, you lose a little of your inhibition, which makes for a great time to try new things.*
> —Amy, 26, Pleasanton, California

Women want partners to connect to their whole person, not just to their genitals. Our genitals are wired to our hearts and minds. One woman said, "Fuck my mind first, during, and after!" Most women need sexual encounters that connect their body, mind, and heart.

☼♡☼ Honey, Come Closer

If men want to penetrate women's bodies, women want to penetrate the psyche of the person living in the body. That is part of what is so hot for women when they penetrate another woman's body, reaching in and touching her on the inside. The physical penetration can also be emotional penetration and takes on a much deeper meaning when you touch the whole woman.

Sex and Emotional Release

Often during sex, whatever emotions have been lurking just beneath the surface will emerge, because when a woman's genitals are stimulated, so is her heart and psyche. People aren't always consciously aware of what's happening to them emotionally as they have sex. Your lover may have an emotional response during sex that neither one of you immediately understands. These emotions can play out in different ways.

For instance, sometimes a woman will cry during sex, not because she is sad, but because she is feeling an intense emotional release. Sex opens people up for many kinds of emotional release.

> *I've noticed that the only time I can really open up and talk to my lover is during and after sex. I guess sex opens me up to connect in mysterious ways that just don't seem to happen at other times. I've learned to appreciate this, but I also realize how vulnerable it makes me, which means I can't have sex with people I don't feel a strong trust for. If I can't trust myself to open up my feelings with someone, I can't have sex with them!* —Jenna, 28, Fullerton, California

Sex makes people cry and laugh and giggle. Laughter is another important and powerful release. When joy, love, happiness, and bliss are on the surface, some tears might be shed, somebody might break out in uncontrollable giggles and laughter, or she might get lost in gazing into her lover's eyes, sharing sweet affection. These are all simply responses to the emotions that sex has aroused.

Emotional Floods

When the darker emotions of grief, anger, or humiliation are dormant just under the skin, they will also be released. If a woman is feeling anger, she might express this by digging her nails into your skin, fucking with a sudden forcefulness or roughness, sobbing, or total shutdown. It's part of the release. Remember, sex is one of the greatest releases, so we let go of whatever we've got that needs releasing when we have sexual contact. Getting rid of the tension in our bodies and lives is healthy!

It can be confusing or even scary if your partner has this kind of emotional response during sex and you don't understand what it is. If this happens, stop the activity. Explain to your partner that you are feeling her anger, or grief, and discuss what it may be about. See if she wants time to herself. She may want to be held quietly for a while, or maybe she needs to yell, scream, and let it out.

When we have genital contact we are also getting heart contact, if we are open. Women are often more emotionally open and available because they are given permission to be emotional by the culture, unlike most men. Women have permission to feel emotion and express it—permission to cry, to grieve, to open up and pour forth. That doesn't mean all women do. But it can make lesbian sex a more connective experience.

Sex can be just physical for both men and women. Fucking can be a lot of fun—it can be a thrill to get with someone and dip into our animalistic urges and just fuck. Slap bodies and fuck and suck and rock and ride. When you are connected everywhere, you can still fuck and get down and dirty, but the sexual experience becomes richer. If you are not receptive by nature, it has a direct effect on your capacity for pleasure. It also affects your ability to pleasure your partner.

> *Basically what I think makes a good lover is emotional and psychological presence. It really is not so much about "technique." If a person is really present and open as a lover, they will automatically be able to pick up cues from the other person and assimilate them into lovemaking.*
> —Sara, 34, New Haven, Connecticut

Sexing the Whole Woman

Sex is not just about one thing. Sex is about everything. That's what makes it so complex, so difficult, so satisfying. It's not just about orgasm, it's not just about the penis in the vagina, and it can't be broken down into neat categories. Sex involves the whole person: body, mind and spirit. It's never simple. The real foundation of good sex is communication, trust, and opening up your whole self. If women confuse you, you will definitely begin to understand them a whole lot more. The sexual tips that follow will be simple compared to this process.

How Women Work

☀ Her Genitals: Learn 'Em, Love 'Em

I love the reciprocity that is there with women, the intimacy that comes with knowing the other body as you may know your own. —Laura, 22, somewhere in Michigan

Most men hate to admit that they don't know something, especially when it comes to sex. Okay, some of you guys are resident experts and royal appreciators of all women's body parts. For you, this will be a brush-up. For the rest of you, if you want to be able to truly please a woman in bed, you have got to know the functions of the parts you're dealing with. Lesbians have a distinct advantage in this area because they've got the parts too.

Most of you probably have half memories of line drawings and pictures in books that never match your lovers. Very few have taken a course in gross anatomy, where you actually dissect a body, or a couple's workshop, where you are given a guided hands-on tour of the body. For many people, women's bodies are shrouded in mystery.

For starters, understand that every woman is different. Women's vulvas come in a variety of sizes, shapes, and colors. With each new lover you have to find your way as if it were the first time. Thank Goddess!

I love my pussy. We have an excellent relationship. I've always been aware of her, and curious, from a young age. We explore together, we respect each other. There's never been a time when I've had negative feelings about her, how

she looks or smells or feels. I care for her health & get regular GYN checkups. We take care of each other.
—Maureen, 41, Brooklyn

Before our little tour it's important to stress what this chapter is not about. It isn't about committing all the names of parts and their spelling to your memory. It isn't about being able to ace a hand-out quiz where you identify the various parts with arrows to the fill-in-the-blanks. What it *is* about is getting a working knowledge of women's bodies so you can better pleasure them. The most important thing you can walk away with is a new way of looking at a woman's vulva, a new respect for its power, a new way of seeing the clitoris, and a new way of relating to it. Let's take a little trip down her pleasure trail.

The Vulva: Her Exterior Genitalia

The pubic hair protects the entire vulva. The vulva is what you can see when your lover spreads her legs and reveals herself to you. "Vulva" refers to the collective outer parts of women's genitals, including the mons (that fleshy mound on the pubic bone), the outer lips, the inner lips, the external portion of the clitoris, the urethral opening, and the vaginal opening. Most people call women's genitals "vaginas." The vagina is an internal part of female genitals—the actual canal. There are many more parts involved, and "vulva" encompasses most of those parts.

The Clitoris: Not Just a Pea-Sized Bump

Okay, all guys want to know about the clitoris, the "magic button": how to find it, how to touch it, how to use it to help a woman come. To utilize it for its full power, you need to know the basics and have the right attitude about this miracle organ. Just like dicks, clits come in all different sizes and shapes. And there's more to the clit than meets the eye.

The clitoris is the only organ in men's or women's bodies that

---

:♡: **Honey, Come Closer**

Quit thinking of the clitoris as a little pea-sized bump. It is not simply a little nub that you press like a nuclear-war prompt button, hoping to see a big explosive display. It is actually a whole system of erectile tissue, spongy tissue, muscles, nerve endings, blood vessels, and glands.

---

has as its sole purpose sexual pleasure. Much like your penis, the clitoris has a highly sensitive head, a shaft that likes some lovin', and roots that extend and swell with pleasure. Women's genitals are similar to men's in many ways, and it may be easier to understand them by thinking about your own.

The Pilgrimage

We'll start from the north, at the belly button, and begin to travel directly south. Maybe she even has a little furry bunny trail with which to lead you. First, you should hit the Pubic Hair Zone. Women wear their hair in a variety of ways: au naturel, in big, furry bushes; neatly trimmed and tailored to their pelvis; shaved in cut-out shapes; with a little tuft of hair up top; or shaved completely off for that little-girl look.

Clitoral Shaft/Clitoris Central

Once you are in Pubic Hair Zone, at the north end (the top) of the vulva is Clitoris Central. There are many parts to the clitoris, inside and out. Moving south, your first stop is the clitoral shaft. The shaft attaches to the clitoral glans, much as men's penile shaft connects to their penile glans. In many women, the clitoral shaft protrudes a bit from beneath the skin like a root under the earth. Sometimes it is quite pronounced, and in other women it is not as distinctive and more flat. Be assured, it is there under the skin, waiting to be touched. Generally, it is hairless. Skin without hair tends to be more sensitive than skin with hair follicles growing in it. Keep that in mind.

If you run a finger across the root shaft in an east–west fashion, you will feel the shaft snap back a bit, like a rubber band. There is a ligament there that holds the clit in place and a major artery and vein through which much of the blood flows in and out of the pelvic area.

⟡ Honey, Come Closer

Many women like to have their shaft stimulated more than their actual glans. The glans is often too sensitive, and the shaft is more of an indirect way to stimulate the glans. And it just feels good to be touched! Sometimes it's good to stimulate the shaft first, and as she gets more aroused, begin to touch the glans more directly.

Clitoral Glans and Hood

The glans, or head, of your penis is the most sensitive part. Same goes for the clitoris. The glans is the part most people think of when they think clitoris. Because it is so highly sensitive, it is protected by a hood—a flap of skin that surrounds it and looks very much like a hood over a little head.

Run that finger south along the shaft, and you will come right up on the clitoral hood. Nestled inside the hood is the clitoral glans or head, a hairless round nub of erectile tissue. Yes, we said erectile. Women get hard-ons too! This head peeks out when the clit gets erect. The clitoral glans contains more nerve endings than any other part of the male *or* female body. (For men, if you are uncircumcised, your foreskin is women's clitoral hood. If your foreskin was removed, your glans is exposed and hoodless and may be less sensitive because of the constant exposure.) These external clitoral parts make up the top of the vulva.

Inner Lips

You will notice that two inner lips attach either to the bottom of the clitoral glans itself or to the hood on either side of the glans. They come in all sorts of beautiful shapes, sizes, and hues. Some look like angel wings, some like petals of a flower; some are plump and some are petal thin. Some fold over each other, protecting the vaginal entryway; some are smaller and open easily; while some look like velvet drapery. Some are symmetrical, some are not. All are hairless and pretty sensitive for most women.

For many women, when stimulating the inner lips, you are also indirectly stimulating the clitoris because they are usually connected. Some people consider all this to be part of the whole clitoral organ because it all works together. The parts are not isolated from one another. When a woman gets aroused, her inner lips (and outer lips) will fill with blood and become plumper. Their color will change to deeper reds, purples, or browns because of the blood flow.

Vaginal Opening

Run a finger down the edges of each inner lip. They might extend to the bottom of the vulva, or they might only go about half or three-quarters of the way down. Open them. Inside, more lush, sensitive tissue. Somewhere between the center and the base you should see the vaginal opening. Again, the look of this opening will vary from woman to woman, depending on how her hymenal tissue transformed or healed, if she had any. Some openings will be very simple. Some are puckered up like a rosebud. Some have lips on either side. Some look like a mouth. Many want to be fed. Feed her regularly with yummy, healthy food, and she'll be good to you.

Remember, it is the outer third of the vagina that is most sensitive in women. The vaginal sphincter muscle is right at that opening, and it is strong and sensitive. It can close in powerful contractions, and it can open up like wings.

Urethral Opening

Also within the inner lips, somewhere between the vaginal opening and the clitoris, is the urethral opening. This is where women pee from. It can be high up, close to the clit, or lower, near the vagina. Some urethral openings are tiny, the size of a pinhole, and may not be visible to the naked eye. Others may be more defined, with skin folds around them, so they are much easier to see. Women's ejaculation comes from two very small ducts (paraurethral ducts) that lie on either side of the urethral opening.

Outer Lips

All of this sensitive tissue lies within the outer lips, or labia. The outer lips have pubic hair on them and are sensitive, but usually less so than the other parts. But this does not mean they should be ignored. The outer lips are similar to your scrotum (they form from the same tissue in utero), and you know how your sack and balls love to be kissed, licked, and fondled. Don't forget about the outer lips. They like to be kissed, licked, and stroked as well!

Many of us have heard of the terms "labia minora" and "labia majora," those hard-to-remember Latin terms. Since these terms mean "minor lips" and "major lips," respectively, they are problematic. You see, contrary to what those anatomy-textbook drawings lead us to believe, there is a wide range in how women's lips (as well as their entire genitalia) look. Some women's minor (inner) lips are more major—larger and more pronounced—than their major (outer) lips! The outer lips may be plump and round or more flat with less flesh, while some women's inner lips hang lower than their outer lips, are plumper, and may have many folds of skin. So it is much more accurate to refer to them as inner and outer lips, since they vary so much in size and shape.

Those terms and the stock depictions of lips in most textbooks as being symmetrical, simple, and small have contributed to many women's shame, discomfort, or dislike of their genitalia.

A lot of women—especially heterosexual women, who may never see another woman's vulva—don't realize that women's genitals are as different as their faces. (Lesbians tend to figure that out eventually.) There are women who spend their whole lives thinking there is something wrong with them because their vulva looks different from the one they saw in a book.

> *The first time I saw another [vulva I] was nude sunbathing with my friend. All her stuff was hanging out. Mine's all inside. It looked so completely different than mine.*
> —Rachel, 28, Long Island, New York

Let's Go Inside!

We've discussed all the sights you will see on your pilgrimage around the vulva. We know you like to see, but now come all the hidden treasures you can't see, the stuff that makes women's genitals seem so mysterious.

The Clitoral Legs

Okay, back at Clitoris Central, return to the shaft. Attached to the shaft are two legs. These legs separate and flare out on either side in an upside-down "V" shape. They extend along either side of the vulva underneath the outer lips. These hidden roots of the clitoris are made of erectile tissue, which fills with blood when she gets aroused. As they engorge, they flare out and expand, making the outer lips plumper.

The Vagina

Let's lay to rest some myths about the vagina. First, it's not a wide-open, gaping hole. Neither is it a passive organ, just waiting to be filled by your active member. Far from it. The vagina is actually a collapsed space that expands and contracts when it's aroused and when it is penetrated. Have you ever had a woman squeeze her vagina while you were inside her? If so, you felt the powerful hug of her vaginal muscles.

The vagina is situated inside, with the anus and rectum on the backside and the urethra and bladder in the front. The bladder sits right on top of the vagina, which is why penetration is sometimes uncomfortable if a woman needs to pee. The bladder can be easily agitated.

At the back of the vagina is the cervix. The cervix sort of feels like the tip of your nose. It is the throughway to the uterus. The texture of the vagina is ribbed because it stretches out when women get really aroused. The cervix and uterus pull up and back, extending the vagina by about one to three inches. The back of the vagina "balloons out," creating more space.

> *Some men get it and some don't. I think some men have never taken the time to get to know the entirety of the vagina. And those that have, generally do a good job or can be guided (and are open to being guided) to doing a good job.*
> —Morgaine, 30, Belmont Shore, California

The G-Spot, a.k.a. Urethral Sponge

The G-spot came up time and time again as a point of confusion for heterosexual men and women. Overall, lesbians tend to be a bit more G-spot hip. Here's the down-low.

The G-spot is not a buried treasure somewhere deep in the nooks and crannies of the vagina. You shouldn't have to send out a search party to find it. Most women's G-spots are on the front wall of the vagina, an inch or two inside. Some actually come right up to the edge of the vaginal opening.

So here's the deal. The G-spot is actually the urethral sponge for women. You men should be familiar with the workings of your urethral sponge—the spongy tissue that surrounds your urethra along the length of your penis. It fills with blood as you get aroused, and that gives you a hard-on, and it shuts down your urethra so you can't pee. Well, a woman has the same mechanism. Her urethra runs along the top of the vagina and is also protected by a urethral sponge. In most women, there is an area where the sponge meets the vagina, and that area has become known as the G-spot (named after Dr. Ernest Grafenberg, the guy who "discovered" it).

How to Find Her G-Spot

If you put your index finger just inside the vagina and pull it toward you with a come-here motion, you should feel her spot. It actually feels different in texture from the rest of the vaginal wall. Usually it is raised up a bit and feels sort of spongy. Its size, like everything else, varies from woman to woman. Its pleasure capacity does too. Some women may really like to have it stimulated, some may not care either way, and some may find it annoying if you play with it. All women's pleasure maps vary, but it is a *potential* pleasure area worth exploring for women who like penetration.

⟨♡⟩ Honey, Come Closer

Certain ways of penetrating the vagina will stimulate the G-spot better than others. Fingers are usually better than dicks for this because they can curl forward and stimulate the front wall better. For intercourse, rear entry (doggie-style) positions are usually good because your dick is at a better angle to get the front wall. There are even curved toys made specifically for G-spot stimulation!

Famous Anus

If you continue to move south of the vulva, there is a hot spot between the vulva and the anus called the perineum. Men have the same spot between the scrotum and anus. It is another nice place to stroke, lick, and stimulate. The anus is there, beyond it all, in the nook where the butt cheeks begin. Many a man has had the embarrassing experience of trying to put his penis in the wrong hole, so learn where everything is so you aim right. If the anus is what you're going for, then groovy. If not, she might not react so kindly.

Anuses vary too, so get to know your partner's and your own by using a mirror. The anus is the puckered opening to the anal canal, which is about an inch or two long and leads into the rectum. Most anuses have some hair around them, probably in proportion to the amount of hair on the rest of the body. The outside of the anus and the anal canal are both erogenous zones that many men and women get pleasure from. They also swell with blood when they are in an aroused state.

If you're anal-phobic, getting to know your and your partner's anal terrain might help you overcome your fear. If not, that's your prerogative, but it certainly is a sweet spot to play with if you're open to it and you and your partner know what you're doing down there. Without a doubt, the anal tissue is extra sensitive and should be treated accordingly. There will be more anal discourse in the "Ass-istance for Two" chapter of "The Ins and Outs" section.

The Muscles

There is a complex system of muscles in both men's and women's pelvises, including the pelvic-floor muscle and, on top of that, the pubococcygeus muscle. Commonly know as the PC, this large muscle tightens the rectum and vagina when contracted. Strengthening the PC can increase sexual pleasure and help you guys control ejaculation. In the next section, we'll discuss how you can strengthen your PC.

Her Organic Nectar

Women's pussy juice completely varies in its texture and in the amount she will have at any given time. Some women just produce more than others. Most women produce more or less depending on where they are in their monthly cycles. At certain

:♡: **Honey, Come Closer**

Don't take a woman's wetness or lack thereof to be a definite determiner of her arousal. She might not seem wet, yet could be really aroused by what you are doing to her. At the same time, she could be really gooey and wet, and it could be for reasons that have nothing to do with you! It could've been the movie she saw an hour ago, a little fantasy she entertained, or simply where she is in her menstrual cycle.

times of the month, depending on ovulation and hormonal levels, she will produce greater or lesser amounts of her special blend of organic femme nectar.

Sometimes you will turn her on and she will quickly respond with hot, wet arousal. Yum. Just do not use her level of wetness as an absolute arousal barometer or pressure her to be wetter for you (unless it's part of some kind of teasing role-play). Lesbian women sometimes pressure each other this way, as if one partner's amount of juice should match the other's. Not fair game. Know that each of your partners will be different from one another and they will vary according to their cycles. If her pelvic muscles are inactive, this can also affect how quickly her vagina lubricates—the more active the muscle, the more lubrication it will produce. Use extra lubricants if they're needed, and don't get personally offended.

Vulva Appreciation

This has been a generic road map to some terrain you may encounter. Now it's up to you to explore the dynamic landscape of each partner's vulva. They are all different and beautiful in their own way, and each has its own unique capacity for pleasure. If you do not know much about women's genitals or are afraid of them, do yourself a favor and learn more by checking out some of the following resources or other publications. The more exposure you have to women's genitals, the less foreign or mysterious they will be. Later in the book, we'll give you some ways to learn about her love muffin. Remember, we all want our genitals to be appreciated, so compliments go a long way. The genitals are our most private and sacred body part. Practice some vulva appreciation, and that vulva and her owner might show *you* some! Tell her how beautiful she is!

♡ Other Resources on Women's Genitals

A New View of a Woman's Body by the Federation of Feminist Women's Health Centers

An amazing book with more details on women's anatomy, for those of you interested in further research and drawings.

Femalia by Joani Blank

Photographs of vulvas. The women are of different ages, races, and ethnicities, and the styles, sizes, and proportions of their vulvas vary too. This book is not like girlie magazines and will give you a whole new take on women's "femalia."

Sex for One: The Joy of Self-Love by Betty Dodson

Betty Dodson is a sex educator and artist. Her drawings of various vulvas (all done with live models) alone make this book worth getting. It is chock-full of information on her work with women, teaching them about their genitals, masturbation, and how to have orgasms.

Viva La Vulva (video) by Betty Dodson

A video about women and their vulvas by this dynamic sex educator. It is the only video of its kind and will be helpful for both men and women who watch it and listen to women talk about their genitals, show them in their various shapes and sizes for the camera, and demonstrate female genital massage.

Zen Pussy (video) by Annie Sprinkle and Joseph Kramer
The only one of its kind, this video is literally a concentrated meditation on eleven different pussies. An innovative new way to release tension and relax.

Fire in the Valley: An Intimate Guide to Female Genital Massage (video) by Annie Sprinkle and Joseph Kramer
This vulva-positive video gives thorough instruction and demonstration of female genital massage. Hosted by sex educators Annie Sprinkle and Joseph Kramer, it discusses the benefits and encourages partners to explore the power of the Fire in the Valley.

See our Resources list at the end of the book for information on where to get these books and videos.

☀ Goin' with Her Flow

If there is one part of women's physical workings that is completely misunderstood by most men, it's their menses. Yet menstruation is totally natural. Many men fear it or are just plain confused by it. Here's a little primer to help you with your lover's period as it pertains to your sex lives.

Sex with a Goddess

Picture a mesa at dawn, tinged pink by the awakening sun. Gathered in a circle are men and women, adolescent boys and young girls, toddlers and babies in their mothers' arms. The mood is solemn yet celebratory; this is clearly a sacred occasion. Into the circle a young girl of twelve or thirteen years is led by the elders, and with great ceremony and dignity she is introduced, first, to the entire community and then to the rising sun. The occasion is the celebration of the girl's first menstrual cycle. Among the Navajo people, this is one of the most important and joyful rites of passage, for the tribe and for the girl whose newly awakened womanhood is being honored.

The Sunrise Ceremony not only marks the first flow of blood and fertility of a young woman; it introduces her to her family and tribe as someone to be treated with a new level of respect. Imagine if you had grown up in such a community, where all boys are imprinted with the understanding that the monthly cycle of a woman is a special and sacred occurrence, not a "curse" or disability. Imagine, as a guy, how you'd feel about menstruation if the blood from a woman's first cycle was captured and ritualized—used to fertilize the crops that would feed the entire community, male and female, young and old—rather than as a vaguely distasteful, unhygienic, or even shameful thing to be hidden from polite company. It would be quite a different world, would it not?

Often the unease has nothing to do with men. In our culture, it often comes from women, because they've been so inundated with negative attitudes about their blood. There is much misunderstanding, shame, silence, and fear about women's menses in both men and women. Men seem to have a particular aversion to and fear of menstrual blood, probably because their associations with blood are very different from women's. It reminds many men of war and pain, whereas women see it as part of their everyday lives, their body's natural cleansing mechanism, and their monthly death-and-rebirth cycle.

Menstrual blood is natural. It's not unclean, and it doesn't equal war and suffering. (Although some women do get pretty severe menstrual cramps and PMS symptoms, so be nice! They are real!) For many lesbians, it's not such an issue, because they are used to seeing their own and their lovers' menstrual blood. Most experience their own version of PMS, so they can empathize. Many heterosexual women's discomfort with their blood is linked to the discomfort (real or imagined) of their male partners.

Pro Choice: When the Moon Is Between Her legs

I am absolutely fine with having sex while on my period. It's kinda messy, but not a turn-off for me at all. I am turned off by lovers who think it's gross.
                              —Sherri, 29, Washington, D.C.

I am uncomfortable having sex during my period, just because it's messy. I also feel a lot less attractive when I have my period. I think that a guy wouldn't be into it either.
                              —Judy, 21, Amherst, Massachusetts

Sex during menstruation is a personal preference, even among lesbians, where both parties have intimate, lifetime familiarity with the process.

I'm a little reluctant, but I can transcend it with a little encouragement. And I like to take measures to minimize the messiness, like putting a towel on the bed.
                              —Fletcher, 52, Charlottesville, Virginia

I don't mind having sex when someone is having her period. But I've had girlfriends who were reluctant.
                              —Beverly, 24, New York

Even those who choose to continue sexual activity during the moon cycle have their own boundaries or taboos. Some will have vaginal intercourse but forgo manual or oral stimulation. And some think this is one of the most amazing times to have conscious, intentional sex.

Having sex on my period is interesting. Sometimes my orgasms are longer and stronger.
                              —Jasmine, 19, Clemson, South Carolina

Some women, of course, are physically sensitive at this time to the point of discomfort. Feeling in the skin is heightened, and

> :♡: **Honey, Come Closer**
>
> Since this is an inherently powerful and heightened
> time, a time that is potentially sacred and magical, it
> would be a shame if you never explored menstrual sex
> just because of cultural prejudices.

the vagina may be swollen or lacking in cervical fluids. For
them, this time may be better spent in the pursuit of emotional
bonding, cocooning, soothing bathing, or pampering. But don't
assume that your lover won't enjoy menstrual sex just because
the two of you have never tried it.

> *We do it all the time. If we're in the mood, we're in the*
> *mood.*   —Melynda, 22, Holland

> *I didn't enjoy sex during my period until I learned to use*
> *my diaphragm in place to stop the flow.*
>   —Gingerbee, 58, San Francisco

Sexing with Her Flow

The "Ooh, gross" mentality surrounding the blood and dis-
charge itself is always a bit befuddling. What do you think
comes out of you, dude, crème caramel? Nah uh. Thick or runny,
opaque or clear, odorless or smelling like the mushroom section
at your local farmers' market, semen is an acquired taste. And so
is menstrual blood. But honestly, you might find that if you give
it a chance, a little flow can be an incredible sexual turn-on. Her
body's natural scents are totally heightened. Going down on her
when there's flow is also a matter of taste and safety. Some
people love it, and it turns others off. Menstrual blood is often
sweet or slightly metallic in taste—all that iron. If you don't like
the taste of the blood, you can concentrate on her clitoral glans
and shaft, staying away from the flow around the vagina. Your
saliva will help the mix spread around as well. The presence of

blood is a bigger risk and safer sex should be practiced unless you have another arrangement.

> *I was a little touchy about oral sex during a woman's period, but I tried it at my lover's request and it was fine. I didn't go as deeply with my tongue.* —Bob, 31, Boston

Part of the problem is that men have always sneaked peeks at "grotty" sanitary napkins wrapped like mummified remains in toilet paper and stuck down at the bottom of the bathroom wastebasket. The fact that these were probably mom's or sis's soiled napkins added to the gross-out factor. But some people get turned on by that sort of thing. Menstrual blood is a rather terrific lubricant, quite silky and fluid, although it can get sticky. Once you're inside her the sensations are amazing! Every nerve is on alert, and the extra lubrication, combined with all that supercharged sensitivity, can make plain old intercourse a whole new pleasure.

> *If there are two times when I'm exceptionally horny and ripe, it is when I'm having my period and when I'm pregnant. I've had sex both ways, and I can tell you, there is a kind of single-minded biological imperative coursing through a woman's body when her hormones are telling her it's time to find the cutest, strongest, smartest cave boy or girl around and get down on the sabertooth skin.*
> —Karen, 31, San Diego, California

༼☼༽ Honey, Come Closer

Slipping fingers, a dildo, or a cock into a flow-moistened pussy can be a tremendously sensual experience for both parties. The wildly sensitive tissues of your lady's insides, the exaggerated feel of swollen labia, and the sweet smell are as much of an aphrodisiac as anything that costs $12.95 and comes out of a bottle at your friendly neighborhood sex shop.

Blood Bond

I love the taste of my lovers' menstrual blood. The problem is that I know it's risky unless it's under specific conditions with a partner who I trust and who has been tested for STDs. It is so intimate to share that part of her, so sweet . . . it really gets me hot to go down on a woman who is bleeding.   —Amelia, 32, Bronx, New York

Maybe the best thing of all about menstrual sex is the bond of trust and intimacy it can create between partners. A woman has traditionally been made to feel unattractive and unclean during her period. The man who gently and lovingly heals that cultural shame is a man who deserves the title "dream lover."

I love sex during my period. It feels good, and sometimes it makes my cramps go away! As long as my partner is okay with it. It really makes me happy.
                    —Terri, 21, Austin, Texas

➡️ **Ten Things You Can Do When the Moon's Between Her Legs**

1. Have a long kissing session.
2. Give each other a massage.
3. Masturbate together.
4. Stimulate her clitoris with your tongue and/or hand.
5. Vulva love: Embrace the Goddess with all her flow.
6. Pearl necklace: Stick your penis between her breasts and go to town (use plenty of lube).
7. Butt slide: Using plenty of lube, slide your penis between her butt cheeks and slip and slide away.
8. Explore toys, toys, and more toys.
9. Anal sex: Explore a new orifice, or visit an old friend.
10. Vaginal intercourse: Let the flow be with you.

The number one reason for treating her to some pleasure while she's got her moon is that *orgasms relieve menstrual cramps,* which makes for much better moods too. You will get more bonus points for cramp relief via some sweet orgasms than for any other single act. It sure beats a prescription of Motrin or disabling naps.

Just be safe about it. If you are not sharing bodily fluids (fluid-bonded) with your partner, remember your latex barriers. Blood *is* risky if your lover has an STI. If you *are* fluid-bonded (have shared bodily fluids), the taste can be oh-so-sweet. It is all part of the nectar of her body.

☀ Orgasm: Be Loud, Be Proud

While definitions of sex varied dramatically among the lesbians and heterosexuals we spoke to, one element seemed to be pretty universal: Sex involves orgasm in some way, shape, or form. So let's devote some time to this stimulating topic.

Left in the Dark

Men have endless questions when it comes to women's orgasms. Actually, *women* have endless questions when it comes to women's orgasms. Unfortunately, orgasm is a phenomenon plagued with confusion, misinformation, and invalidation for the better part of recorded history.

Most of us spend a lot of time in our formative and later years trying to figure it all out. Most people get a sense of satisfaction when they bring sexual pleasure to another human being, and we want to know how we can best do that. We want to have mutually satisfying experiences, full of joy, pleasure, and orgasms! You wouldn't be reading this book if that didn't matter to you. We hope that a lesbian perspective will clarify some of the myths and help you make sure her orgasm is an integral part of your next sexual liaison.

The Mythical Story of O

Once upon an orgasm there was Sigmund Freud, who put out some ideas that truly did women a disservice when it comes to orgasmic pleasure. Freud stated that in women, vaginal orgasms are "mature" orgasms, while clitoral orgasms are "infantile"—only for masturbating little girls. He helped promote the false idea that the vagina is women's sexual pleasure center and thus, women should have orgasms through penetration of their vagina. We now know this is erroneous and that the clitoris is actually women's center o' pleasure, but it takes time to snuff out widespread myths, and this one has burned brighter than a long-life bulb. Many heterosexual women think something is wrong if they aren't having orgasms through penetration. Lesbians don't have the same pressure. To this day, many women still want to "learn how" to have "vaginal orgasms," but the vagina doesn't have enough nerve endings for orgasms to occur without some clitoral action. There are so many parts to the clitoris that it's always involved.

Men got gypped with Freud's vaginal myth too. Here are all these men, trying so hard to get their female partners to come solely from penetration, and when they don't, the men think they are doing something wrong, or that their partners must be frigid. Any man who is huffing and puffing, trying to get her to scream in orgasmic ecstasy from thrusting alone, might make her feel good but won't necessarily make her magically climax in wild penetrative abandon. History has taken its toll.

☼♡ॢ Honey, Come Closer

Men, it does not mean you are a bad lover if your partner does not reach orgasm through vaginal intercourse. It does mean that the two of you need to explore clitoral stimulation and other ways to get her hot. Also, don't think that because a woman doesn't reach orgasm through vaginal intercourse that she does not enjoy penetration!

I had a lover who had discomfort with the intensity of having an orgasm through sex that involved penetration. However, she was very comfortable with orgasms through receiving oral sex. To her, penetration required a different level of trust to really let herself go.
—Maggie, 25, Yonkers, New York

Many women totally get into some in-and-out lovin'—in a couple of different orifices—even if they don't climax that way. Conversely, there are women who don't like penetration at all, in which case you will really have to expand your ideas of what sex is and work with each other so you can both get your needs met. This doesn't mean you have to give up penetrative sex altogether, but you may have to negotiate a little how you will fuck.

Teamwork

In my experience, the difference between sex with men and sex with women is that with women, we aren't done until we both *come. There's more of a mutual feeling about it.*
—Danielle, 31, Syracuse, New York

We discussed how the clitoral glans and shaft are analogous to the penile glans and shaft. Can you imagine having sex and never having your penis touched except by accident? Would you be unfulfilled? If it happened over and over and you never had orgasms, how would that affect you? Would you get frustrated? Bitter? Angry? Would you still want to have sex with that partner? Far too many women speak of having partners with no clue about how to find a clit, how to approach it when they do, or what it's for. Enough is enough.

Some women do not have orgasms. This is not because they can't have them. It might be because they haven't learned how. Any healthy woman can have an orgasm if she learns how her body works. Then it's up to you to do your part and make sure her clitoris gets some action. For many women it can take some time. Orgasm doesn't magically happen after five minutes of cli-

> :♡: **Honey, Come Closer**
>
> To have orgasms with your lover requires teamwork. Encourage her to teach you what turns her on, just as you need to teach her what you like. Otherwise, you'll be blindly searching for the key to the kingdom. Communication and trust will help her open up and share her pleasure with you.

toral sensation. You need to take time with her and care whether she gets satisfied.

To a large degree, it is her responsibility to communicate what she wants, what feels good, and how she needs to be touched and stimulated to reach orgasm. Then you have to put into practice all that she's told and showed you (since it's probably different from what you did with your last partner). In an ideal world, both partners would do their "part." Some women have a lot of experience with pleasuring themselves and know just what they need. Others have been more dependent on their lovers to figure it out.

Since we don't live in a perfect world, you'll need to know what you can do to put your lover on the orgasmic path and avoid the road that leads to a non-orgasmic dead-end.

The Orgasmic Richter Scale

> *My last orgasm was the fullest, richest, open-nosed orgasm I ever had. Like it took a lifetime of fucking to get to that point. We discussed it afterward because my wife had a comparable orgasm . . . though not simultaneous.*
>
> —Richard, 50, Berkeley, California

All orgasms were not created equal. For anyone. Sometimes we have a nice little bunch of localized muscle spasms in our pelvis and we think, "Ah, that's sweet." Other times it feels as if our pelvis will rupture from the rapture. Then there are those incredible full-body orgasms that spin into our head and numb out our hands and feet in tingling ecstasy. Beyond that, we have out-of-body orgasms that feel like they might send us through the roof, or leave us spinning in a dizzy euphoria, ready to greet the light. There are so many kinds of orgasms. We can't have an out-of-body spiritual experience every time. Sometimes it takes a lot of work to cultivate the powerful energy that creates such ecstatic events.

> *My orgasms aren't very great, but they are satisfying. In-stead of muscle contractions, I have a warm feeling that is usually concentrated in my pelvis and abdomen, but some-times it reaches down to my toes. Getting five or six in a row is best because the last one will be the strongest and most satisfying. I would like to improve my orgasms, but I'm very busy right now and it's fairly low on my priority list. I'm not worried because I know I can always improve sex if I devote some time to it.* —Rebecca, 40, New York

In women, there have been distinctions made between orgasms that are clitoral/vulval, vaginal/blended, or uterine. The Federation of Feminist Women's Health Centers' excellent book *New View of a Woman's Body* redefines the clitoris as an entire organ and the central structure of women's sexual anatomy. With this "new view," they deduce that *all orgasms are clitoral.* This revolutionary idea would render any debate over clitoral versus vaginal orgasms moot. Yet women do report experiencing different types of orgasms and that they do feel different from one another. That's probably because different parts of the clitoris get utilized. Whether or not we call all orgasms clitoral, the importance of the clitoris is certainly indisputable.

Multiple Orgasms

So what's the deal with multiple orgasms? What does it even mean? Definitions vary, but basically it means being able to have a few in a row, pretty close together, without a refractory (resting) period in between or only a very short one. The pattern can vary. You can have a bunch of little ones, or a couple smaller ones and a really big one, or a huge explosion followed by twenty "aftershocks." It may seem like a volley of rapid-fire orgasms, or you may take a short break, then come again soon without needing to roll all the way back down the hill. However they come, they keep on coming!

> *My clitoris needs to be stimulated just right and it creates*
> *the highest climaxes. I climax progressively higher and*
> *higher each time until—after three or four orgasms—I can*
> *reach the ultimate place that moves me out of this plane*
> *and into another dimension. Relaxation, security, and a*
> *close emotional bond help bring me to climax.*
> —Roz, 52, south Florida

Part of the reason women can keep riding the wave and have orgasm after juicy orgasm is that they don't have a depleted erection to overcome. Of course, like men, they often reach a point where any more stimulation is just too much. Outta this world. So let her rest—all her nerve endings are standing on end, and she may need to relax a minute or ten. But if she wants to work toward multiple orgasms, the trick is to keep going, maybe pause a minute, or put a hand under the vibrator to diffuse it a bit, or focus on breasts or something else a moment, then boom! Get right back into it, push her over the hump, and continue the orgasmic response.

Female Ejaculation and the G-Spot

Yep, that's right, some women ejaculate. The better question to ask is: What's the big deal? Female ejaculation has been so suspect that even doctors and other "authorities" have refused to document it as a valid phenomenon, even though it has been part of recorded herstory dating all the way back to Aristotle!

The G-spot is pretty consistently linked to ejaculation. Women usually ejaculate when their G-spot is stimulated through the vaginal wall. Sometimes when there is a long buildup to orgasm, women will ejaculate without any G-spot activity, but usually the G-spot is involved. Women will ejaculate a healthy amount of fluid that is different from the cervical and vaginal fluids that lubricate the vagina and often leaves a little puddle.

The best way to stimulate the G-spot is with fingers or a curved toy that can reach the vagina's front wall, where the G-spot lies. It is possible to stimulate it through intercourse, but certain positions will be better than others. The phallus is at a good angle for hitting the G-spot for many women when doin' it doggie style, or in a woman-on-top position, where she can control the angle better. If she leans back a bit in a sitting position while you lie on your back, she can get her G-spot stimulated. One woman reported that adding abdominal pressure with her hands while in this position helps her partner's cock hit her in the right place.

> *My orgasms are definitely of a different quality. While masturbation and oral sex are great, my best explosions are when she is on top and my ankles are around her ears. This always has a guaranteed result of having to change the sheets or at least needing to put a towel down first.*
> —Mari, 26, Marina del Rey, California

You could end up with a sizable wet spot. Some women even squirt! If you are worried about the mess, just put a towel underneath her. Sex towels are always a good thing to have on hand.

Your Reaction to Her Ejaculation

Lesbians tend to be more G-spot and female-ejaculation savvy than most folks. We haven't heard of many lesbians leaving—or being really grossed out by—their partners because they squirted. On the contrary, it's usually more a call for celebration. The level of comfort and knowledge most lesbians have with the female anatomy and its orgasmic mechanisms contributes to that. When people get upset over female ejaculation, it's usually because of their false assumption that it's pee.

> *I'm proud to say I've been with two women who've ejaculated. It is fascinating to watch and extremely intense, and it is definitely not pee.* —Karen, 24, Queens, New York

Alice Ladas, Beverly Whipple, and John D. Perry are well-known researchers of female ejaculation and the G-spot. They have noted that ejaculation seems to be more common in lesbian and bisexual women than it is in heterosexual women. They note two possible reasons why this might be true: "Perhaps, as with the G-spot, it is sometimes easier to reach the area of sensitivity with a finger than it is through penile contact. Or, perhaps, females may be more accepting of the fluids expelled by other females than males seem to be."

Their tests and examination of the chemical makeup of female ejaculate showed that it is not urine. Some researchers call it female prostatic fluid, proposing that there is a female prostate gland. This ejaculate comes from two glands on either side of the urethra.

Whether a partner is open to a woman ejaculating can determine how positive the experience is or if she will even do it at all. If she is feeling embarrassed or thinks her partner will not re-

:♡: Honey, Come Closer

If you make comments about her ejaculate smelling or soaking your sheets, you could cause her embarrassment, make her think there is something wrong with her, or that it's gross or unnatural. These thoughts may cause her anxiety during sex. This will make her hold back in the future so it doesn't happen again. If you react supportively, encouraging her to let go, or if you really like it and it shows, she will feel good and confident about ejaculating. Then she can further explore that part of her orgasmic response.

spond favorably, she may well hold back and not fully let go, fearing her partner's reaction. Most of this has to do with changing the perceptions about women's ejaculation, getting people to understand that it is a common orgasmic response different from urinating. If your lover ejaculates while sexing it up with you, your reaction can cause her either shame or pride.

Enhancing Orgasmic Pleasure

Raise Your Voice for Orgasms

Sexual vocalization, no matter what the volume, is one of the sweetest sounds in creation.
                                   —Eric, 22, Roanoke, Virginia

Some people feel comfortable moaning loudly or screaming with wild abandon when they reach orgasm, and others never allow themselves to do that. There can be something pretty hot about having a silent orgasm because your parents are in the room down the hall or because you don't want to get caught. Being forced to be silent can heighten the intensity of the fantasy and the release. But if you make a habit of retaining sound rather than releasing it, you may be depleting the power of your orgasms. Try letting it go. When you release all the mechanisms involved in the orgasmic response, you fully experience your orgasmic capacity.

♡ Honey, Come Closer

Silence can really stifle an orgasm. By not allowing your own sound to push up and through you along with the muscle contractions, blood flow, and heavy breathing of the orgasmic response, you cut it off. Sound is a primal release and, for many, a big turn-on! What better sound is there than your lover screaming, moaning, crying out, or singing her own ecstatic song? Encourage her to sing!

His and Her Workouts for Better Orgasms

In the genitals chapter, we mentioned the PC (pubococ-cygeus) muscle. Both men and women have one. A major or-gasm muscle, the PC is like any other muscle in your body: when you work it, it gets in shape, increasing in strength, en-durance, and efficiency so you can do more with it. For women, a strong PC muscle is also vital for childbirth, making for an eas-ier labor.

> ### :♡: Honey, Come Closer
>
> Some women report having orgasms for the first time after strengthening their PC and beginning to activate it during sex!

Since I have been exercising my PC muscles, my orgasms during sex have been more intense because my body seems to be more involved. My last girlfriend was actually im-pressed with my muscle strength.   —Rachel, 31, Chicago

The PC muscle runs from the pubic bone around to the tail-bone (coccyx). In men it runs underneath the testicles and around the anus; in women, it runs underneath the outer lips and around the anus. Let's practice locating it. Ready for some light calisthenics?

It's the muscle you pull up on or contract when you want to stop the flow of urine midstream. Try pulling up on that muscle now. If you have a hard time finding it, go and urinate and stop it midstream and you should be able to figure it out. Okay, time for the workout. Here we go . . .

And pull up, *hold,* one . . . two . . . three . . . four, okay, re-lease. Again, pull up, *hold,* one . . . two . . . three . . . four, okay, let go. And one more time, pull, one . . . two . . . three . . . four, and let go. You are now doing Kegel exercises, named after the gynecologist who popularized them. It's really helpful for both men and women to do this simple exercise. When your pelvic muscles are toned, you will have stronger orgasms, and people who have never had an orgasm may learn how by starting to work the muscles. A major part of the orgasmic response is the tension that is released from our muscles.

For women to work the muscles even more, believe it or not, there are actually vaginal barbells on the market, called Kegelsizers. The Kegelsizer is a sleek stainless steel one-pound barbell that women can insert into their vagina while they do their PC reps. The barbell gives the vagina something to contract around, providing resistance for the muscle. Kegelsizers aren't cheap, but luckily they double as a nice dildo for women who enjoy penetration. Any good sex shop will carry them. A relatively thin dildo will also work; watch as each rep pulls the dildo further into your partner's pussy and then releases it.

You can do Kegels anytime. The more you do it, the stronger the muscle will get. The best part is, you can do Kegels anywhere and nobody will even know! You can have a little workout each day or a few times a week while riding in your car, waiting in line at the bank, sitting at your desk at work, dozing through a boring staff meeting, having lunch with a friend, or relaxing at home. Do thirty, fifty, or one hundred reps each time. You can also vary the time you hold each rep—do some for an eight-second hold, then quick pulsing reps to practice a quick response. If you have a partner who is not having orgasms or is unhappy with her orgasmic response, having a little PC workout together can help you both.

The Role of Breath

Breath is a very important yet often forgotten part of arousal and orgasm. Deep breaths enhance the flow of energy throughout our bodies, and the more that energy is moving, the more you can do with it! It's easy to forget to breathe. Many of us can recall a sexual encounter where we or our partner's face got red and contorted, and they pulled back fiercely, not breathing, just pumping away like a marathon runner about to reach the finish line. Breathe, child, breathe. Breath distributes oxygen, nourishing the blood that is racing through the body. Not only does it help the blood flow; it gets more of the body involved. Holding your breath can stymie your orgasm in a limiting way.

Sometimes holding your breath can intensify sensation, but it should be done consciously, not because you're forgetting to breathe. Some people like to hold their breath as they bear down into the orgasm to help bring it on. That's called auto-asphyxiation.

If you have not consciously worked with your breath during sexual arousal, try it. Experiment with your breathing and see how it changes your arousal pattern, your buildup, and the length and amount of your orgasms. Yoga and the Tantric discipline both work with the breath and its effect on the energy of the body. Working with your partner to synchronize your breathing during sex may enhance your connection.

You also want to work your breath with your PC contractions. Try breathing in and pulling up on your PC, hold, then let both muscle and breath go simultaneously. Then switch it. Pull up on your PC on the exhale. See the difference, and figure out what works best for you. Just remember to breathe, and remind your partner too!

Arousal

What's the measurement unit for women's orgasms, or is there one? How can you tell when a woman has one? Did she have an orgasm or not? Should I stop licking her pussy or keep going? She didn't scream like my last partner did when she climaxed, so maybe she didn't. How do I tell?

For many men, a woman's sexual response can be confusing or unclear, especially since different women are going to experience and express it in various ways.

The stages of sexual arousal in men and women have been widely documented by sex researchers. Depending on the point of view of the researcher, the stages are divided up slightly differently. During these stages, a woman gets a hard-on just as you do. Her package fills with blood and swells, her inner lips perking up, plump with pleasure. Her clit swells and gets erect. She gets wet. Her vagina expands. Her muscles tense, and as they release, she has an orgasm, even ejaculates, and if stimulation ceases, she slowly loses her hard-on and everything eases back to its usual resting state.

The stages overlap and vary in length and intensity from person to person, but the basic sequence and pattern remain the same. People's experience of these phases is much more subjective and fluid than the well-known academic model. Having a set of stages is a pretty linear way of looking at such a complicated and widely varied mechanism as sexual arousal. It is important to remember that arousal has emotional, psychological, and sensual elements as well. It's not simply about genitals. Try to understand what actually happens in her body throughout her entire sexual response. The crucial thing is feeling it with your body and recognizing it in your lover so you have an understanding of the basic changes that are likely to occur and the range of women's bodily responses during sexual arousal and orgasm.

> *Sometimes I can tell that my partner had an orgasm by the rhythm of her movements, and her breathing, as well as the contractions in her vagina. Sometimes it's hard to know, especially if you're not paying very much attention. Sometimes it helps to hear "I'm coming . . ."*
>
> —Ace, 29, Guadalajara, Mexico

The Basic Journey

When you and your partner start to get aroused, both of you are warming up the entire body. It's kind of like the first quarter of a basketball game: You're getting a feel for the game, finding the rhythm, the flow. It's like the beginning of a story, when you are getting to know the characters—in this case, yourself and your partner.

The first prickles of excitement begin in the mind. This could

> ☼♡ **Honey, Come Closer**
>
> Sexual arousal has a pattern: a waking, a building-up, a rhythm, a singing, a crescendo, a slowing down, a stillness.

be triggered by almost anything: smells, sounds, seeing the one you love or some other erotic image. This starts hormonal changes in the body as testosterone and estrogen are released. It could be set off by something as simple as gazing at your partner or holding her hand. In simple terms, you're getting horny.

You are kissing, stroking, fondling, exploring each other's body, playing in the excitement of being together. Your mind is entertaining all sorts of naughty fantasies. The action starts to build, thickening the plot and the blood flow in the body. This might cause a skin flush, where the skin changes color. You start to sweat. In a woman, blood rushes into the vulva, filling all the erectile and spongy tissues in the lips and clitoral parts. The clitoris enlarges and becomes more sensitive.

Maybe you've slowly undressed each other and you're standing in the middle of the kitchen floor. The combination of fondling, kissing, and seeing each other naked has become too much. She grabs something and so do you—and we're not talking about a saucepan. You clear the counter in one fell swoop and spread out, or you go horizontal on the linoleum.

As the action intensifies, the body moves into a more heightened state, like the suspense in your own personal movie. As they fill with blood, her breasts enlarge slightly and her nipples become erect. The vagina releases a lubricating fluid. The outer lips draw back and the inner lips swell. The inner portion of the vagina expands, while the front third swells with more blood, tightening. The color of her vulva will deepen to shades of crimson, purple, or brown.

As you can see, so much happens before you even get to

what most men consider the actual sex action: thrusting, sucking, fucking. Let's say you are diligently diddling her clit with a well-lubed fingertip, hissing hot words in her ear as she grips your oiled cock in her tight fist, milking the shaft with wild abandon. As the pleasure mounts, so does the tension, and you both experience the muscle contractions as waves and peaks of hot and luscious sensation. All this stimulation inches you both closer and closer to climax.

Remember that men and women are more similar than different. Many of the same things happen in their bodies. The breath rate and heartbeat increase. Intense sensations begin to build in the genital area. As the breath deepens and the intensity of the feelings increases, a series of wavelike muscle contractions in the genital area build to a crescendo, and there might be an expulsion of fluid as your head spins, your body tingling, as you go over the top into bingo—ORGASM! The Big O.

Each basketball game and each story has a different ending. Some are emotional and intense. Others are light and funny. And not every sex session has to end with orgasm. They can be chapters in an epic novel.

You've reached a climactic moment, whether it included orgasm or not, and you are both sated. You slow down, decrease, or cease stimulation of body parts. You relax in each other's arms and conveniently grab a cookie (since you're already in the kitchen) or order takeout to quell the appetite you've worked up. Within a couple of minutes her vagina shrinks back down to its resting state; the clitoris and uterus relax and return to their usual positions—the clitoris in about twenty seconds, the uterus in about twenty minutes. The muscles are warm and relaxed, and you have that healthy afterglow.

Okay, guys, now you know the drill. Having a better idea of these bodily changes, the flow of desire, and how to identify the physical mechanisms of her pleasure will make you a better lover—if you become responsive to them. This doesn't have to make the process mechanical. Remember, there is no such thing as the perfect kiss, blow job, or fuck. And there is no such thing as a perfect way to experience arousal. It all depends on you and your lover's pleasure and connection, and what you hope to explore.

Understanding arousal is about opening up your awareness. Ultimately, the best experts in the world are you and your lover. This knowledge is a tool. Every story has a beginning, middle, and end, but the good ones are still full of surprises along the way.

Orgasmic Recap

The world of arousal and orgasm is so vast that anyone who puts conscious effort into expanding their orgasmic capacity will see results. Hundreds of variables affect our orgasms: the mood we're in, how much mental and physical energy we have, whether we are masturbating or with a partner, how much we like our partner, how present we are, breathing, working our PC, fantasizing, how much we can let go, the type of stimulation, where we are, how comfortable we are, what turn-ons we need. Be conscious of her pleasure and response, and happy cumming!

It's All
Play

☀ Foreplay? Honey, It's All Play!

Most folks have their own little barometer indicating when foreplay ends and sex begins. Definitions vary. For most heterosexuals, foreplay seems to be everything up until a penis enters a vagina. For lesbians, foreplay can be anything leading up to actual touching; for some, the concept does not even compute.

> *I believe that foreplay is a misogynist concept, centered on male access and orgasm. It's about preparing the woman for intercourse. Foreplay as a concept is genito-centric and goal-oriented, which is as much a drawback for men as it is for women. For me, it's ALL sex, different aspects of sex, which may or may not lead to orgasm, but which is all-pleasurable and all-inclusive. "Foreplay" implies that you're "getting ready" for the "real thing," rendering everything else as "less than." The concept of foreplay totally relegates lesbian sex to the status of "not-sex." This applies to much of heterosexual sexuality as well.* —Robyn, 40, Brooklyn

♡ Honey, Come Closer

Here's a little secret: It's all play. From the way you hold her hand, gaze into her eyes, and snuggle next to her, the way into a woman's heart and pants is not a paint-by-numbers procedure (kiss, play with her tits, rub her clit, then give it to her).

Most of you guys have been educated to think of the sex process as a kind of isolated mechanical process: Foreplay starts with a kiss and ends with penetration. The biggest gap in this way of thinking is neglecting the psychological and emotional part of sex, which involves communication and touching that is not goal-oriented. Who decided that sex is only a penis in a vagina? Who decided that a vast world of possibility is diminished to one act, everything else becoming secondary, mere lead-up to the real pinnacle of heat—penetration?

For many heterosexuals defining sex as something other than intercourse is a virgin idea. That's why so many men are curious about what lesbians do in bed. For lesbians, this idea can be pretty offensive. You try telling a whole group of sexual women that all this sweaty, wet exploration of skin, breasts, lips, and orifices is not sex. See if you get out of the room alive. Oral sex is sex. It even has sex as part of its name, just like vaginal sex, anal sex, manual sex, and sex toys.

> *Foreplay begins with talking about how you feel—words are extremely powerful and very attractive—then all the general flirty touchy things, and then maybe you can think about it being time to kiss her neck.*   —Fish, 29, New York

Many people consider kissing one of the most intimate acts and consider it part of sex. Others disagree. Maybe it depends on the context, but if a person calls kissing sex, then it's sex.

You need to start looking at your entire sexual interaction as play. Sex certainly takes on rhythms: some sweetness, a slow pace, glances, nonverbal suggestions, caresses, kisses, building up, getting hotter, faster, more intense, with more body parts involved, possibly orgasmic, until, at some point, a slowing down, a resting, a stillness. It's up to you how you write the song, how long the verses last, how much you free-style and improv, how it builds, how it ends. Sex does not have to be a linear 18-hole course. It can be much more natural than that if you only learn to follow your impulses, your gut, your feelings. Do what feels good, and get feedback from your partner on where she wants to go. Open up your world!

If you are looking at all the preliminary proceedings before "intercourse" as "foreplay," then you miss out. Men often have the tendency to focus on getting to intercourse, only going through the motions with everything that comes before it. Great sex means being fully present in each moment of a sexual encounter.

It can make a person feel vulnerable or hurt to have sex with a partner who is not fully present. Women will pick up on that. They know when their partner isn't there with them and is merely going through the motions to get to what s\he really wants. This is the fastest way to alienate, confuse, or lose a partner. Don't do it. Learn to slow down and enjoy your lover. Take in the fullness of her body, of how it feels with yours, of her responses, of your responses. With all this orgasm talk, we might forget that good sex can happen without seeking orgasmic release. Spending time feeling your partner's body, kissing and hugging without feeling pressured to reach orgasm, can be satisfying in and of itself. Many lesbians prefer sex that is not goal-oriented. The following chapter in this section will give you specific tips, helping you tune in to the process of making love, making it all play.

☀ Tune In to Her Senses

You have a powerful little sex army working with you to create the fullest, most powerful assault on her body! This special battalion is your senses. If you are not using them at all, or are only tuning fully in to one or two, you are crippling your sexual experience and power.

Men are known to be visual creatures. Women are known to be verbal creatures. That's how the stereotype goes. But we bet there is a whole lot of variety in the ways people get off, and they're not based on our assigned gender! So if you tend to just use one or two methods to turn your lover on, try to incorporate others to see how much more balance and pleasure you can achieve.

Gazing, Peeking, Admiring

The ancient Greeks believed love entered through the eyes. Gazing at your lover's body, creating a visually stimulating atmosphere like a dreamy, candlelit room, watching her dance or undress, watching some erotic porn to get the two of you in the mood, or "reading" a hot magazine together are all ways we deploy our sight brigade in sex.

You're a man. You like to look. It's probably gotten you into trouble before. You've stared, ogled, done a double take. You've commented on a woman's build and been called a pig. There is commonsense etiquette when it comes to gazing at a woman: no shouting out numbers from one to ten, no catcalls or whistling in public, no stupidity. Don't stare at her breasts or ass for an extended period with your mouth hanging open or that stalker look in your eyes. Don't size her up from head to toe, looking at everything except her eyes. Don't forget that part of looking at a woman is making eye contact. This doesn't mean you shouldn't adoringly gaze at women, appreciating their bodies and beauty. Some women may not want that kind of attention, but many of them also love to turn heads and be looked at, especially when it's done respectfully.

> *One of the hottest things a woman ever did to me was tie me to the bed and erotically dance for me. Although I was blown away and I couldn't really function, it was quite a sight to see.*   —Christy, 29, Port Chester, New York

The one who'll appreciate you watching her the most is your partner. Don't be shy. As long as you don't embarrass her in front of other people, you can actually whistle and make catcalls at your lover when she looks hot—she'll probably find it flattering and playful. Get some of that staring and ogling out of your system with her—she'll love you for it. Gazing at the one you're with is not only a turn-on, it can also create emotional connection and build trust. Know every inch of your lover's body and face. Gaze sweetly into her eyes when you're with her.

There are many fun ways to raise the visual stakes to enhance your sex life:

- Masturbate for each other.
- Ask her to do a striptease, or just lean back on the bed and watch her dress or undress.
- Watch a porn video you both like, or look at a hot magazine together.
- Be daring and do a Full Monty striptease for her.
- Play "Photographer and Model," and take some Polaroids.
- Make your own home video.
- Maybe you are one of those people with mirrored ceilings or walls. Otherwise, you can use a full-length mirror so you can both watch your own live peep show. One that stands freely can be pulled over in front of the bed, couch, kitchen table, wall, or whatever else you're doing it on. You'll have front-row seats to the hottest performance in town. If you and your partner respond strongly to visual cues, mirrors are a great tool.

Poetry, Music, Whispers, Shouts

Turn her on with your voice. Be sweet, soft, sexy, dirty. Sing to her. Read her a poem. Read her an erotic story. Describe one of your fantasies. What does she like? The sweet, comforting sounds of nature? Listening to the neighbors get it on? The sound of your breath?

> *I really really like talking dirty and hearing it. Words work better for me than photos.* —Cal, 24, Denver

Music is a great mood enhancer and creator. The right music can do wonders for a hot night. On the other hand, having the

TV blaring in the background with mindless programs and obnoxious commercials is not a good idea.

> *I am a very aural person and need to hear my lover's voice,*
> *either talking to me in my ear or screaming in ecstasy. That*
> *gets me off more than anything. I can really get into the*
> *sound, and I've had a series of partners, both male and fe-*
> *male, who all had incredibly sexy and appealing voices.*
> —Jenny, 26, Chicago

Body sounds are another crucial piece. Tune in to the music of your bodies. Tune in to the sounds of kissing, breathing, moaning, and gasping. Listen to all the sweet sounds bodies make together: slaps, slurps, spurts. The body is its own orchestra, so listen and let it enhance your experience and connection to your lover.

Salt, Sweat, Love Fluids, Mangos, Bananas, Honey . . .

Do you like the salty taste of your lover's sweaty body? The sweet taste of her skin? Her mouth? Her neck? How do the various areas of her body taste? Go on a little culinary body tour—it will be fun for both of you.

If you've both been tested for STIs and are sharing fluids, their flavors can be part of the lovemaking experience. What do her vaginal fluids taste like? How do they vary at different times? Does she ejaculate? What does that taste like? Fair is fair.

What about incorporating food into lovemaking? Ever share a sticky juicy mango with a lover? Feed each other berries and whipped cream? Better still, whet her appetite with all sorts of yummy foods for a meal she'll never forget. If you are not a cook, create a romantic atmosphere, order in something scrumptious, serve it up nice, and she'll still appreciate it to her tummy and her mind's content. For bonus points, feed her seductively.

Flowers, Soft Scents, Aromas

Smell is the runt in the litter of the senses. Pushed out by the stronger, more obvious littermates, it is often ignored or underappreciated. Diane Ackerman, in *A Natural History of the Senses,* talks about how we have little vocabulary to describe and discuss what we smell. Well, sometimes words *are* limiting. Smell is a lush world we can dive into without having to qualify what it is we like. A familiar smell can take us to a specific memory of a long-ago time and place. Each person's body has its own unique smell, and that can be the hottest scent on the market. Just be in her smell for a while. Even a little stink can be a sweaty turn-on. We often mask our body's natural smells with perfumes and colognes, and while those might be arousing for some, for others they are distracting.

Smell is our most primitive sense. It has an immediate physical effect that stays in our memories forever. The salty smell of ocean and seaweed, the fresh green scent of pine and flora—the crisp smells of the great outdoors can invigorate you and your lover. Flowers can sweeten any date.

There is no bigger turn-off for women than the gym socks and stale sweaty-guy smell that seems to loom like a thick cartoon cloud in many a bachelor pad. It is to your advantage and her relief to get that stink out of your place and get some good smells going.

The obvious suspects are incense and aromatic oils—you will be a star-quality guy if you keep a little selection on hand. Look for the purest ones; not all incense was created equal. For starters, try jasmine, Egyptian musk, or Nag Champa.

Kisses, Cuddles, Massage

Q: What is your largest sex organ?
A: Your skin.

If you want to really connect to your partner, start by touching her body. Explore it all over, with your hands, mouth, nose— with *your* whole body. There are so many ways to touch. You can caress, massage, stroke softly, sensually, intensely, pinch, bite, pull, stretch, use nails, feathers, spatulas, bodies, and tongue. You can start soft and build the intensity of your touch.

> *I learn a lot about my partner's anatomy by simply closing my eyes and feeling with my fingers and tongue, starting at her toes.*   —Lisa, 27, West Milford, New Jersey

Touch is the base of the sexual landscape, yet it's amazing how many sexual exchanges occur without any real touching of bodies going on. Exploring your lover's body does not mean going straight for her breasts and then her genitals, bypassing the rest of her bodacious parts.

If you don't like to be touched, why? What about it don't you like? Are there certain areas where you really don't like to be touched? What are they, and what do you link those feelings to? Explore your own feelings about touch, and it may help you open up to touching others more if that's something you need to work on.

Post-Orgasm Skin Rejuvenator

A crucial moment to touch your partner's body is after an orgasm. This will help the orgasmic contractions and tingling energy set into her body. Run your hands softly over your partner's front, down her spine and her legs, and along her arms. Caress her head, breasts, and tummy. Stroke her sweetly while the aftershocks and pulsing of the orgasm continue to course through her body and the blood flows furiously through her veins.

> *My first girlfriend had a way of making me feel safe and comfortable enough to let go with her. She would always take me into her arms and hold me right after I came, whispering, "I've got you. You're safe, baby," all the while stroking my body as it tingled. It felt very nurturing and healing, in a way no man had ever made me feel.*
> —Joanne, 29, Dallas

Setting a Mood to Make Her Swoon

Without a doubt, women attach high importance to mood for an appealing sexual encounter. It's not difficult to set a good mood. All it takes is a little forethought, a few items, and some common sense. Obtain some of the staples on this list—they'll do wonders for mood enhancement.

☺ Mood Enhancement

- *Candles, candles, candles.* Lighting is crucial. Or try colored light bulbs for your lamps: Red is sexy, blue is dreamy, purple is passion, orange is warm, black lights are racy, and there are any number of other colors she might appreciate. Start with what feels good to you.
- *Incense.* Get yourself a nice little collection for when you want to instigate some good lovin'. Again, pick out incense that moves you. Musky types are good, or earthy smells. Remember, incense that comes from the purest essences tend to be the best.
- *Sexy music.* Music is a very helpful ingredient in a sexual encounter. Depends on your mood, your likes and hers, but be sure to have some surefire good-lovin' CDs with lots of sexy grooves in your collection.
- *Pillows.* Pillows make for a cozy environment, and they also come in handy for various sexual positions, so you can never have too many on hand. Use them as needed, and toss them off the bed, couch, or love seat when they're in the way.
- *Nature.* A great sunset at the beach, a fresh-smelling mountaintop, the sound of a cool running stream, a bed of leaves, or your own tent anywhere in our lovely Mother Earth's gardens—these are some of the best mood enhancers you will find. The only thing to remember then are the blankets (being

cold does not make for fun whoopy), the condoms, clean hands and fingernails, and a flashlight.

- *Fun food.* Fruit (berries, mangos, and peaches are excellent), hot chocolate, whipped cream, honey, or any gooey, yummy, fun-to-lick-and-slurp food always adds some joy. The physical pleasures of sleep, sex, and food always complement one another.
- *Flowers,* especially large, fragrant ones, are a colorful, romantic touch—provided she has no allergies!
- *A hot bath.* Combined with any or all of the above ingredients, a bath really sets the tone for a romantic, sexy evening. Give her one. Bathe her yourself. Decorate around the tub with roses and candles, sprinkle some petals in the water along with some soothing bath salts, oil, or suds, add some nice music, and voilà! She'll be putty in your hands! Just be sure not to mix too many smells—if they conflict, it's havoc for the nose and the body.
- *A fireplace.* If it's cold out and you have one, there's no better place to cozy up. Fire is always a good passion igniter as you warm up while staring into the hypnotic flames.
- *A Romantic Meal.* There's nothing better to seduce a lover with than the aromatic smells and tastes of a meal you prepare for her yourself. A romantic meal can incorporate all the senses perfectly: the lush smell and taste of spices and comfort food, candlelight, your pretty eyes for her to stare into, hands and feet touching beneath the table, sweet talkin', and soft music. Women are knockouts at providing the sweetest romantic meals for lovers, so do the same for her! Get with it, men. Learn to create a wonderful evening inside, with good food, good music, good drink, and good company.

☀ Kissing: Make Out or Break Out

There are so many ways to kiss: softly, slowly, yearningly, sweetly, probingly, deeply, sloppily, passionately, coldly, dreamily, harshly, passively, demandingly, givingly, penetratingly, shallowly. Some say you can learn a lot about people and their bedside manner by the way they kiss. Some say kissing *is* sex.

♡ Honey, Come Closer

Follow the golden rule: *Do unto others what you would like to have done to you.* Pay attention to the way she kisses you, and return the flavor. In the beginning it's best to play it safe until you know what her tastes are.

Lipmus Test

Is a kiss just a kiss? Just a prelude to a symphony, an appetizer before the main course? According to the women we surveyed (and the men), if the kiss isn't appetizing, there probably won't be a six-course meal! Kissing for most women is crucial, just as important as sex, if not more so. So whether kissing seems very important to you or not, take heed: It will likely be important to your partners. Lesbian women know the power of a good kiss, and of the importance of their mouths and lips.

> *What makes a good smoocher? Wanting it.*
> —Richard, 50, Berkeley, California

To share our mouths, the place from which we speak and through which we feed our bodies and breathe can be one of the most intimate acts: enveloping another's mouth with your own, breathing into her, breathing with her, sharing the same air, sharing saliva. Kissing is a microcosm of the entire sex act. It's the first physical conversation, beyond the small talk and trying to impress her by saying the right thing. Time to get down to business. No more words, just speaking to each other, breath to breath, lips to lips.

> *I love the sensuality that comes with slow kissing, full lips, the closeness of each other's breathing. Regardless of what is going on anywhere else in the body, I can become so connected and rhythmic with kissing. I enjoy deep French kissing, but that is more erotic for me, and I like that during sex more.*   —Shel, 29, New Haven, Connecticut

Kissing is also a kind of relationship barometer. When a relationship starts to go bad, couples usually stop making out before they stop having sex. It's the same reason many prostitutes will perform all sorts of sexual acts with their clients but will not kiss them: they are withholding one of the most sacred acts, unwilling to share that kind of intimacy with strangers.

Male Kissing Death (MKD)

Many heterosexual and bisexual women complain that in the beginning of a relationship men are all into kissing, but once they can "get what they want" when they want it, they seem to forget how to kiss. Don't let this happen to you. Most women need lots of smoochin'. The significance of connecting to a partner through kissing does not dwindle over time. If you don't want her sex drive to dwindle, then keep your kissing drive alive. It was important in the beginning. Make sure it stays important.

> *Kissing is the most important thing. It's usually the first physical step. Soft kisses to start out with. Never French kiss as the first kiss in a series of kisses.*
> —Mary, 28, Cleveland

> *Kissing tells me if she wants to have sex, and tells me what sex is going to be like with her.*   —Donna, 38, Seattle

Elements of a Kiss

There are some basic elements to think about in working on your kissing persona and technique. Kissing isn't something we just know how to do, any more than we automatically know how to change the oil in a car. It takes a good teacher to show us, some practice, and a spark to pique our interest. Whether you've experienced the joy of an amazing kissing partner or not, we can all use a brush-up, so pucker your lips and get ready.

Luscious Lips: Lingeringly and Playfully

Lips are a powerful and magnetic sexual tool. There is nothing like focusing on a beautiful pair of lips, painfully eyeing them all night long—or for months, even years—just wanting to touch them, to wrap your own in their embrace. Lips are incredibly seductive, one body part we can get lost in for days on end. Give in to her lips, indulge them, merge with them, surrender.

Women have soft, sweet lips, perfect for kissing. Most of those lips like to be kissed and paid attention to. So when you do get the opportunity, linger lovingly on her lips. Don't pass up their power in your eagerness to get some tongue. Relax and spend some time with these sensuous organs of pleasure.

Make no mistake about it: Kissing is absolute seduction. Be playful, and create some buildup. Don't make it too easy. Move in slowly for more kisses. Work it, boy!

⚬♡⚬ Honey, Come Closer

Kiss her lips ever so gently at first, then pull away slightly. Putting some space between her lips and yours gives them time to get acquainted. Let her long for your lips. Tease her.

Brush your lips softly over her, ingesting her scent. Allow her to bring her lips back to yours. If, when you move away, her lips are slightly parted, then you know she is wanting more. Gradually get more adventurous. Suck gently on her lower lip, move from corner to corner, a peck here, a nibble there. Start with light, soft kisses, and each time you come back, linger a little longer to build tension. Court her lips and you lay the groundwork for a long, passionate interlude.

> *If a woman can't kiss, I won't take it any further—honestly. I can't get aroused. A good kisser has a good mix of tongue and lips and does not thrust her tongue down your throat.*
> —Barbara, 25, New York

> *I've had partners who weren't good kissers at first. But over time our kissing evolved. We listened with our lips, and we talked about what we liked and disliked.*
> —Jane, 28, Los Angeles

If at first your kissing styles don't match, talk about it. Ask your partner to kiss you the way she would like to be kissed.

Tongue and Mouth: The Dance

Once the make-out session has commenced, there are a few rules that seem to be pretty universal. Keep your tongue in your own mouth until it is invited into hers. If you have to pry her lips apart to get your tongue through, be assured that she does not want it in there. Go slow.

> *Kissing is very important, mostly because it's the first intimate contact you have with a woman and it will inevitably leave a lasting impression. Good kissers don't open their mouths wide open, and they don't just "lock in."*
> —Chris, 29, Mystic, Connecticut

If all goes well, when neither of you can stand it anymore, your lips will part in a breathy, speechless invitation that says,

"Yes, my darling, come inside. Let's get to know each other." Once you have the proper invitation, gently allow your tongue to wander in between her lips, just into the foyer of her mouth. Explore gently at first, and then, as your mutual passion grows, you can probe a little deeper. One thing you don't want to do is jam your tongue down her throat. That not only can be an unpleasant invasion, but might even be startling for her. Always work up to deep French kissing. Just as you took your time with her lips, slowly and gradually explore her tongue and her mouth.

Think of it as a dance. Your tongues are engaged, moving together, moving apart, teasing a bit and coming back again. Keep in step with her. Your tongue shouldn't be too overbearing, smothering hers. Give her room to breathe. Don't do the locked-jaw two-step. On the other end of the spectrum, you don't want to be darting all over her dance floor, never following through with the last step, either. It's a good idea to share the lead with her. You can lead a little, then you can follow hers and see how she likes to dance. Flow with her, and if the passion builds, you might end up totally sucking face in a crazed frenzy of dirty dancing.

Communicate all the way with your lips, mouth, and tongue. They speak volumes, so say it with a kiss and make sure you are saying what you want her to hear. Remember, it's the ultimate litmus test and should leave a lasting impression.

Taste and Smell: The Intimate Exchange

At such close proximity, the kiss is our first taste. As you run your lips over hers, even kissing other parts of her face, you get the first savor of her skin and lips. And don't forget to take a sweet deep breath, appreciating the nuances of her smell. Many of the lesbians we interviewed spoke of the scent of a woman as a major reason for her attraction. The smell of skin and the taste of lips and mouth can be irresistible, unforgettable.

A good kisser is tender and curious and doesn't rush. Little tastes and bites, teasing nibbles. We taste each other's breath.
—Curtis, 45, New York

If your tongues end up intertwined, you will also taste her and she will taste you. Hopefully it will be appetizing and keep you coming back for seconds and thirds. Savor her flavor like your favorite dessert. Just mind your manners and avoid slurping and slobbering.

> *Good kisses require good mouth hygiene, my confidence,*
> *and feeling safe. Kissing feels more intimate than inter-*
> *course to me.*   —Joanie, 51, Fort Lauderdale, Florida

It goes without saying that bad breath is a total turnoff and won't get you to square one of the kiss—or anywhere else, for that matter. Be an attentive lover and take the necessary precautions so you don't have a bad case of halitosis to contend with. She'll be disappointed, and the kiss will surely suffer. You want to taste good for her.

Rhythm

> *Kissing is the most important thing both before and after*
> *sex. It gives me an idea of how relaxed the person is, it lets*
> *me smell them, and it lets me see how good we are at fol-*
> *lowing each other's rhythms.*   —S.J., 36, New York

Perhaps one of the most important aspects of a kiss is the rhythm of the dance. Kissing is music in its sweetest form. Think of the variety of rhythms in music and liken them to kissing. Kissing can take on the long, lingering notes of a sultry jazz ensemble, the erotically charged excitement of flamenco, the fast-paced, hard fury of a metal riff, the stops and starts of an alternative song with constant tempo shifts, the steady, deep beat of African drumming, or the sweet simplicity of a three-chord folk anthem.

If you are an intuitive and inventive kisser, your rhythms are going to change from day to day, with your various moods and with different partners and their moods. Many people have a certain rhythmic style they generally stick to, but it will change depending on circumstances. You don't want to get programmed like a top-40 song that gets boring fast. Your ability to flow with your partner and adapt to her rhythm will make kissing more fun and engaging.

> *Kissing is everything! A kiss can tell you a lot about how the person is in bed. Someone who tries immediately to match your rhythm is someone who is most likely attentive in bed. Someone who thrusts their tongue down your throat or slobbers is inattentive or inexperienced (respectively). I find that kissing is the most romantic and passionate part of any sexual relation. A good kisser is someone who varies in their kissing: they may nibble, suck, bite, match your rhythm, initiate their own. . . . A creative kisser is the best kind.* —Beta, 22, Detroit

⚝ Honey, Come Closer

Change it up. Don't get stuck in one staccato rhythm that painfully repeats itself over and over like a bad techno song. As the desire between you and your partner shifts, it should express itself through your kiss. You can be creative by exploring the many aspects of the kiss. Vary your rhythm between long, slow, deep kisses and quick, light, whimsical ones.

Passion and Energy

All technique and puckers aside, at its core, kissing is an intimate exchange of energy between people. You might have the technique down to a science, but if you have a new smoochin' partner and your combined energy is off, the kiss will be too. Sometimes it's just the way it is. It's no fault of either party, but the energy and passion just aren't there. The pheromones aren't kicking in, and neither is the rapture.

But when the energy exchange is electric and alive, those are the kisses that will have you seeing your version of fireworks. The sexual and sensual energy in both your bodies will get a jolt, and the power of it all will combine and intertwine in a passion-filled kiss you won't soon forget. Your lips, mouths, tongues, and entire bodies are having an intense conversation.

Use your hands to gently explore: Hold the back of her neck, stroke her hair, or hold her hand. Remember that a deep kiss is the time to engage your body with hers in a dance. Pull her into you so she can feel your passion. If you press into her, heart to heart, chest to breast, warm bodies nestled so close, you might both fall into uncontrollable rapture.

> *Kissing is important to me because you can tell how a girl fucks by how she kisses . . . and how bad she wants you to fuck her or if she wants you to go away. . . . A good kisser, hmmm, wet and probing but not too intrusive, maybe "questioning" is the better word.*   —Chrissy, 31, New York

Finding Your Own Style

Everybody has his or her own style of kissing. Many people will liken the way you kiss to the way you make love. You want your style to have some flair, something that makes it uniquely you. Hopefully this will just happen naturally. It shouldn't be something you think too much about.

> *There's no such thing as a good smoocher. It's a good match of styles. If both people's styles work, blending together, that makes for a good kiss. Nothing is more awkward than incongruent kissing.*
> —Kitty, 21, Westchester County, New York

So many elements go into your style: the way you move, the feel of your skin, the texture and size of your lips, how you wield your tongue, your level of attention, how much you care about your partner's pleasure, how much you like your partner, how much you like yourself, your confidence level, how aggressive you are as a lover, your sensuality, and how much you enjoy kissing. All these things will play a role in your style. Some of them can be changed or shifted; some can't. You will surely start off on the right foot by placing kissing in high regard and paying attention to your lover.

> *A good smoocher is someone with whom you can create your own individual style of kissing. No two people kiss alike, and you have to tell your partner just what it is that you like doing and having done to you.*
> —Jasmine, 18, Clemson, South Carolina

Advanced Kissing 2000

There are, of course, infinite combinations of these basic elements and hundreds of ways to kiss. You can create a sampler plate of your own. The following can get you started or extend your kissing portfolio.

Two on One

Usually a kiss is lip to lip. But sometimes it's nice to mix it, giving one of your lover's lips a little extra attention. Just make the bold move and capture and caress either her upper or lower lip between yours and focus on that lip. Give it a little suction, move it in and out between your lips, even give it a little nibble. If you do it to one of her lips, don't forget to give the other a little special lovin' at some point. Now, be fair!

The Light Touch

Sometimes it's a nice change of pace to leave her lips and explore the landscape of her face. A good kiss for this expedition is light and dry, tenderly contacting her skin, then moving on to the next destination, always leaving her wanting more. Lightly explore her whole face with a hundred love kisses so she knows how much you appreciate one of her most personal body parts.

Full-Body Kisses

Kissing isn't just for the lips. If you are getting into various stages of undress, do it with a kiss. Hands, feet, fingers, and toes all love to be kissed and sucked, as does the back, all the way up and down the spine. A soft tongue running along the length of the spine, doing little circles around each vertebra, is incredibly stimulating, sending pleasure signals directly to the brain. And don't forget belly kisses, inner-thigh kisses, soft kisses on soft breasts, and swirling, suction-filled kisses on hard nipples.

Tongue Curls for the Girls

The value of tongue technique cannot be overestimated. It is obvious that jamming a tongue down a woman's throat is not a popular act. What you want to do is get creative with your tongue and have some fun. A tongue curl is just what it sounds like. To try it, stick out your tongue. Now curl it back toward your mouth in a slinky, inviting dance move, like you're luring the object of your affection to you: "Com'ere, baby." That's the motion of a tongue curl. You can explore the various nooks of your partner's mouth with tongue curls. A little to one side or the other. Or curling slowly or briskly along the top of the mouth. Curling with her tongue in a cha-cha-cha will keep it interesting and flows much nicer than the dead-weight tongue we mentioned earlier or the overeager manic tongue most women would just as soon do without.

May the Force Be with You

Literally sharing your breath—your life force—is a truly intense way to kiss, immersing you completely in your partner. Once you are engaged in a deep passionate kiss, use this to up the ante or sweetly end the kiss. It works best with a partner whose rhythm you are able to match without missing a beat. It requires complete focus.

First, you will need to lock in, mouths open and tongues still, then simply breathe together rhythmically. As she exhales through her mouth, you inhale the air as it is released, then send it back, then suck it in again. It may take a little trial and error to get this right, but when you do, you are essentially creating one beating heart where your bodies become chambers working in unison. You will end up breathing slightly in through your nose so as to bring fresh oxygen into the mix. It's not something you will do for extended periods of time, but it can be the sweetest way to cap off a memorable kiss, connecting deeply, sharing life force, mouth to mouth, lung to lung.

Use Your Hands (That's What They're There For)

Good dancers gracefully bring their hands into the mix. How aggressively you use your hands depends on your bedside personality and how well you know your partner. Just get them out of your pockets and put them to good use. You can hold her hands, stroke her hair or her cheek, gently squeeze her upper arms, rub the back of her neck, run your fingers up and down her spine, squeeze her butt, pull her hips into yours, lightly brush against her breast, stroke her hair, or gently pull or tug on it as you nibble her neck.

Always start easy with hair tugging. For some women, it can be totally hot to have their hair pulled to reveal the neck, which is promptly devoured with some of your smoochin'. This can be a complete turnoff for other women, so you might want to have an idea first whether she'd be into that or not. Whatever you do, avoid inducing any whiplash, or you will be the one getting whipped, dear.

Quiet Lips

Here's a little Zen kissing exercise. Just press your lips together with hers and don't do any smooching movements. Try
to feel your entire body in your lips and in your connection.
Then take a moment to let your hands explore each other as
your lips stay connected and still. When you can't stand it any
longer, wait another second, then one more second. Then break
out into some more activity.

Vampire's Kiss

The neck is absolutely crucial for passionate kissing. We all
have a tender area that runs from the bottom or back of each ear
down to our collarbone, on top of the shoulder. It's called the
sternocleidomastoid (SCM) muscle, and sticks out a bit when
our neck is arched to one side. You don't need to remember
what it's called, just where it is. When it's kissed, sucked, and bitten just right, chills will rush up your victim's whole spine and
fill her head with a swirling euphoria.

Biting isn't just for vampires. Of course, timing is again of the
essence. This type of kiss can't come out of nowhere. You've got
to build up to it. Once you're getting into the throes of a long-
lasting, passionate kiss and you move from her mouth to her
neck, wait for the perfect moment when she arches her neck so
you can better kiss it and gently bite her SCM. Don't hurt her!
Sort of grip it between your teeth tenderly. You don't want to
break the skin, and you don't want her to scream out in pain.

This can be a good time to try a little hair pulling. Give her
hair a gentle tug, and it will expose her neck so you can suckle
it. If you do it just right, she will shiver, giggle, sigh, or moan passionately and keep her neck open to you. You can nibble and
suckle all along the sensitive SCM. Now be fair and get the other
side. Be careful, though—most people don't appreciate hickeys
(not visible ones anyway). Don't give her one unless you know
she gets off on that sort of thing.

When done gently, vampire love bites can feel good not only

on the neck but also on the lips, ears, upper arms, butt, breasts, thighs, tummy—almost any fleshy area. Just don't bite too hard!

Ear Suckin'

Next stop: ear suckin'. Some people don't like it. But again, if you do it proficiently, she'll be candy in your mouth. Be careful when you suck on her ears. Avoid making squeaking sounds that will send distorted hi-fi into her brain. Total turnoff! Be gentle yet firm. Suck the top of her ear, kiss it all around. Suck on her earlobes. If she's wearing earrings, they can be cumbersome; just work around them and avoid swallowing them. If you go for broke and decide to stick your tongue in her ear canal, do it with style, do it sweetly. Don't just stick it in there and give her a wet willy. You'd better be talking as passionately with her ear as you were a minute ago with her mouth. Don't get it all sloppy wet. Chances are, she won't like a sloppy kiss in her ear any more than she will in her mouth. Remember, go easy on the saliva. If you do tongue her ear, blow lightly on it immediately after. It will feel cool and tingly to her. Breathe in her ear. Lightly moan or whimper sweetly. She's listening. You're right there, so express yourself with sound.

Prelude to a Kiss

Okay, now you're an expert kisser. So how do you smoothly get over that intimidating hurdle of the first kiss? Let's talk.

Kissing is all about timing. Since it's part of the main course, you need the kissing equivalent of a cocktail and a scrumptious appetizer. This might be giving her a little hug and a kiss on her cheek when you say hello. If you do this, your chances of getting more at the end of the evening increase dramatically, providing, of course, that the date goes well. It shows you are suave and debonair, a perfect gentleman. Lesbians make wonderful gentlemen. Follow their lead. A kiss on the cheek is harmless and sweet.

> ### ☼♡☼ Honey, Come Closer
>
> The key to setting up a good kiss is not waiting until the end of the date to start touching. Lesbians touch and hug all the time. This makes the transition to kissing much easier.

After this initial contact, find ways to keep it up. Touch her arm or hand while you talk. If you feel daring after a little arm contact, graze her thigh. Let your legs accidentally touch and linger for that extra moment, then steal away. These are little kissing appetizers. Don't do anything to freak her out, and don't let these little moments of contact go on for too long. Most important, pay attention to her reactions. This is interplay, not one-way play. Be aware of the give-and-take.

You're engaged in a flirting game. You're building trust and physically breaking the ice. You're brightening each other's dimmer switches. All these little actions are paving the way for the first real kiss. If you've done the work to build up to it and the perfect moment presents itself, be ready to act.

Psych yourself up before the date. Mentally prepare. Say to yourself, "If that great kissing moment arises, I'm going to seize it." If you do, you will be in her Kissing Hall of Fame forever.

Going for It: The First Kiss

Being Rhetorical

Some men like to ask first. If you're unsure or you feel it will make your date feel more at ease, then by all means ask. In an ideal world, "Can I kiss you?" should be more of a rhetorical question. It's best to propose this question when the woman is posed in your arms and her lips are parted, waiting for yours. She should be so overcome with desire that she can barely respond. The only thing she has left to do is lift her head a little higher to meet your lips.

Kiss Me, You Fool

Just grab her impulsively and plant one on her. This is daring but not dangerous. All she can do is say "no thanks" or turn away. And if she does so, respect her choice and don't let it devastate you. Sure, it will be awkward for a minute, but the minute passes and you move on.

This moment is really more about preparation than spontaneity. Most of us have experienced or imagined the perfect kiss. The world slows down. You are looking into each other's eyes, and all you can think is "I want to kiss her." You pull her into your arms and see excited passion in her eyes. You lock gazes, find her lips, and plant a sweet, light peck on them. You pull back to look into her eyes again. They tell you all you need to know. If it's there, you begin the intercourse that kissing is.

What If the Kissing Sucks?

You need to be honest about the make-out session. If it just doesn't feel right, don't push for more by projecting things that just aren't there. And don't push it just to fulfill the need to get laid. If your kissing styles and tastes don't match, it's wise to take a step back and evaluate. Maybe the two of you should just be friends.

> *Kissing is so important. I just went out with a guy who couldn't kiss at all. . . . It was like kissing the palm of my own hand. I knew as soon as he kissed me that we would not be together for long. A good kisser doesn't slobber, doesn't choke me with his tongue, doesn't move immediately from kissing me to grabbing my crotch. . . . A good kisser sees kissing as erotic for its own sake, not a means to an end.*
> —Suzanne, 29, New York

On the other hand, although it's very important, kissing doesn't have to be the be-all and end-all. It certainly makes sense to give things a chance to evolve. Even though we like carrots, we can also learn to like peas. We may need to give some time to learning the erotic rhythms of a new partner.

Kissing, after all, is a matter of taste. There is no objective, universal, perfect way to kiss. The perfect kiss depends on the likes and dislikes of you and your partner and on the energy between you. So if the two of you aren't clickin' in the kissin' department, talk about it. Tell your partner what works for you and what doesn't. If you like each other enough, this conversation could put you on your way to building a longer-lasting relationship (or at least getting a second date) if you can get over the awkward hump. You have nothing to lose by trying.

Rules for the Kiss to Make the Ladies Swoon

Sometimes people kiss and it's electric, like the kiss they've waited for all their lives. Other times there's just nothing there. It's intangible. It's about energy. It's just the way it is. But if you follow these helpful lesbian rules of tongue, you won't completely blow it.

1. Be present, be present, be present. What does that mean? You've got to be there. If you kiss like there's nowhere in the world you'd rather be at this moment in time, like the rest of the world doesn't even exist, you will be 75 percent home. Really. This means don't kiss in a rush to get your dick somewhere. Or while going over your taxes in your head. Kiss for the simple, pure essence of kissing in and of itself.
2. Be passionate. If you don't understand this, go back to rule number 1.
3. Don't slobber all over the place. Wet, sloppy kisses are sometimes a good thing, but go easy, especially when you are getting to know someone. It's like anything else. Err on the side of caution on unfamiliar terrain. If she hates sloppy kissers and you lick her like a melting ice cream cone on a hot summer day, you're gone.

4. Relax and go with your instincts. Explore her. Court her. Get to know her with your lips and mouth.

5. Your tongue shouldn't lie there like a dead fish. It should be active. There's nothing worse than having to search around for a kissing partner's absent tongue.

6. Don't ram it down her throat either. There's nothing wrong with deep, wet kissing. Lots of women like it. Just be sure to build up and create a rhythm. Start slow and gentle, smelling her, tasting her with some little nibbles on her lips. Acquaint yourself with her mouth first, and then you can work into more pene-trating, deep, luscious, or wild kissing.

7. Find your own signature kissing style. There is no formula. Kissing is your soul peeking out and reach-ing for hers. If you're afraid, she'll feel it; if you're shut down, she'll feel it; if you are open and yearn-ing, she'll know it. Kissing is a grand communication of feeling or the lack thereof.

8. Variety is the spice of life. Mix it up. Most important, ask your partner what she likes. Ask her to kiss you the way she likes to be kissed.

Creating Your Own Language

Kissing is communication. It's a body conversation. It's a will-ingness, an openness, a spontaneity, the ability to listen, to re-spond, to control or not control, to surrender, to not know, to discover, to die and be reborn, to rise again, to grow tired, to find a second wind. It's a gesture, a voice that can express irony or understatement, prove a point, lay down the law, tell a joke. How sloppy? How much pressure? How much tongue? Kissing is the way you dance and move. It's the full expression of who you are. Put your whole body and soul behind your kiss.

SMOOCH!

☀ What's Best for Breasts

After the initial burst of charm, most men concentrate on "getting on first." There's usually a relentless race to second base, followed, often too quickly, by the "quest for the rest." While this might win you a sandlot championship, it will not put you in the Great Lovers' Hall of Fame. We hope by now you're already rethinking your strategies when it comes to the dance of love. You're mastering the fine art of teasing, remembering it's *all play*, working on your communication skills, and—yikes!—surrendering to the idea of emotional involvement. As a reward, let's spend a little time luxuriating in the rolling hills and gentle valleys of the territory known as the Land of Breasts.

Real Breasts: Like a fingerprint

Just like the vulva, breasts and nipples come in many different sizes, shapes, and colors. In our culture it's nearly impossible for a woman to feel good about her breasts. They're either too big, too small, or not a full, symmetrical C cup. Hence, the world of Wonderbras and implants.

> *My breasts cause me so much anxiety, because they are so out there for everyone to see and judge. So I wear a padded bra and dread the moment when I have to undress in front of a new lover.* —Jerri, 23, Baltimore

Passing the Test

To add insult to injury, there's the old pencil test. It goes something like this. The woman stands topless in front of a mirror and places a pencil under the lower crease of her breast. When she lets her breast go, if the pencil falls to the ground, she's perky; if it stays she's saggy.

Imagine a male version of the pencil test! "Gentlemen, hold

that same pencil alongside your penis. If your penis does not reach the eraser, you're inadequately endowed. Sorry!"

I remember this guy I dated laughing hysterically at the "tit shots" in National Geographic. *It made me never want to undress in front of him. I mean, that's how real breasts look when they are not pushed up by a Wonderbra. Tits have to obey the laws of gravity just like everything else in the world.*   —Tracy, 30, New York

Here's the point. Put yourself inside her bra. Lying back against the cushions on the sofa, the subject of your desire has been exploring the possibilities of sexual compatibility with a man—you. She may barely know you, or she may know you well but not intimately. You've passed that awkward moment when the thought of sex has turned into kissing. Hands have been held, lips have met, tongues have entwined, and mutual rapid breathing has begun. So far, so good! Suddenly, a hand strolls down her shoulder, making the descent to her breast. This is when her blood pressure begins to rise, because she knows that the foray into breast territory leads to the removal of clothing and she fears that the soft rolling hills of her landscape won't live up to your expectations. She is about to do the dance of vulnerability for you, removing her clothes while you sit fully dressed, your own potential inadequacies zipped away.

I guess you'd call me large-breasted. It makes me very self-conscious. The first time I undress in front of a new lover, I want to make sure he sees me standing, not lying down with everything flopped out and hanging over the sides.
          —Maggie, 29, New York

Like most sexual dilemmas, the best answer is usually pretty Zen: Be here now, stay in the moment. All those other true clichés apply, particularly for the underappreciated netherworld of "second base." Forget about getting below the waist while you're hiking the Tetons, grand or small, and just enjoy them.

Unveiling Like a Work of Art

Like a sweet lesbian lover, your sense of style when undressing the breast sets the stage for everything else. Shucking it out of its bra cup like an ear of corn won't leave her impressed with your finesse, dramatic sense, or timing. A man who spends time exploring the breasts from the outside shows patience and confidence rather than desperation. This may sound silly to you, but a lot of women carefully pick out their undergarments to arouse you, and it is disheartening if you simply rip through them. And just because a woman isn't wearing a bra doesn't mean you should go right for her breasts. Teasingly stroke them through her clothing, then slowly work your way underneath, touching all around them, moving in closer and closer. Touch her breasts briefly, go away, then come back. Remember that these are just guidelines and variety is important. Making a beeline to her breasts and fondling them like your very life depended on it can also be exciting.

> ### ː♡ː Honey, Come Closer
>
> Make a dance out of it, so the lovely orb is revealed with grace. If you take time to appreciate each layer, she'll appreciate you. Make it a moment. Take off one strap at a time as you kiss her shoulder and gently caress her breasts, then unclasp her bra and take it off ever so slowly. Be playful about it and take your time.

Breast Etiquette

Some women like it when their breasts are touched lightly and cringe when they are squeezed. Others like to have their breasts kneaded and firmly squeezed. Some women like it when their nipples are nibbled, pinched, and clamped. Other women writhe with pleasure when their nipples are stroked with light feather touches. And some women will not like breast play at all. Their breasts are too sensitive; breast stimulation simply doesn't feel good to them, or discomfort with the size or look of their breasts can inhibit their getting any pleasure out of them. It's the same mantra: Everyone is different.

> *My breasts and nipples aren't very sensitive. It's not a primary area of stimulation for me.*   —Terri, 27, New York

Breasts are as diverse as penises when it comes to roughness or tenderness. Even though you see it in a lot of pornos, pinching and twisting a woman's nipples is not a major turn-on for all women. With nipples, it is especially important to communicate. A squeal is hard to interpret. Is it pleasure or pain? If you're not sure, ask. There's a fine line between pleasure and pain; make sure you walk on the pleasure side of it—unless, of course, she's into rough play. A little pain is exciting and fun when both partners are into it.

Until you find out what she likes, go slow, read her body, and follow the cues.

> *I don't like pinching or biting right off the bat.*
> —Lindsey, 27, San Francisco

> *I like gentle nibbling.* —Bobbie, 25, Aberdeen, Washington

> *I don't like my breast squeezed like a cow's udder.*
> —Liz, 24, Queens, New York

> *I like lots of sucking, pulling, and squeezing.*
> —Maggie, 26, Brooklyn

> *I like a little nibbling, not too rough though. In long-term relationships there have been times when rough biting was fun. Hickeys on the breasts are fun.*
> —Christine, 31, Waco, Texas

Let your fingers do the walking before you presume to get oral. It's best to introduce yourself to her breasts with gentle fingertips instead of homing in madly and sucking on the nipple like a starving man. Take your time with her breasts. This will make her feel appreciated and help put her at ease with you.

Sometimes a man just gives one of my breasts love. That's an insult. You're saying I don't even want to be here long enough to give both your breasts the time of day.
—Carol, 39, Oklahoma City

Give each breast equal time! Alternate from one to the other. Set up a rhythm between the two just as you create a rhythm on one.

❀ Honey, Come Closer

Bring one breast to the point of heightened arousal by feathering and caressing her with your fingertips, and just when she's sure you're going to press your lips to her nipple for a suck and a swirl, slide over to the other breast, leaving the first panting for your return.

The Nipple: Nature's Little Thermometer

Okay, it's nipple time. Men love hard, erect nipples. So do lesbians. Hard nipples equals horny, right? Not always. She might be cold or nervous. Erect nipples are a beautiful thing, but don't interpret them as a surefire sign that she's hot and horny and ready for intercourse. It's also important to understand that the nipples and breasts enlarge in the days prior to a woman's period. At this stage of her cycle they may be extra sensitive. So don't take it personally if your lover asks you to go easy. Her breasts will desire different things at different times of her cycle.

When I'm PMS-ing, I hate to have my nipples touched.
—Laura, 26, Cambridge, Massachusetts

Since the nipple is nature's thermometer, why not use this sensitivity to your advantage? Different temperatures evoke different sensations with breasts. Ice cubes have a powerful effect on nipples. Rub your lover's nipples with ice, then surround them with your soft lips for some warm sucking. Or try a warm massage oil on the nipple or a cooling peppermint oil, then blow softly.

☼ Honey, Come Closer

A great technique is to wet her nipple with some sucking and licking, then blow on it so the cool air makes the nerve endings contract. This can be a very pleasurable sensation. And don't think it's uncool or not macho to enjoy the same kind of play and pampering with your own handsome titties. Allow her to return the favor and discover the extent of your own nipple sensitivities.

Let's Hear It for the Areola

Just as the vagina often becomes the immediate or even sole point of focus for the sexually clueless man, so the bud of the nipple tends to get all the attention. If the areola didn't have such strong self-esteem, she might have some issues. This lovely and sensitive pigmented tissue surrounding the nipple is filled with pleasure-giving nerve endings. Her areolas may be generous or nearly nonexistent, shell pink or latte dark, but regardless of size or color they are the launching pad for a thousand subtle reactions. In fact, the area around the nipple tip may be far more wildly sensitive than the bud itself, and deserves its fair share of attention. Make sure you give this encircling ring, this heavenly halo, plenty of love.

I love it when a lover laps her tongue all around the bud of my nipple, so my silver dollars get all hard and tight.
—Kim, 28, Austin, Texas

And don't forget those little bumps around the perimeter of the areola. They are tiny hair follicles and are exquisitely sensitive. Yes, unlike *Playboy* centerfolds, some women have hairs on their nipples. Run your finger lightly around the circle of follicles. Nipple-areola stimulation can send shudders all the way to your lover's clit.

I can have orgasms through breast play.
—Ingrid, 32, St. Louis, Missouri

ː♡ː Honey, Come Closer

An encounter with the breasts is more like the first stage of fellatio, where a skilled woman will tease and tantalize you to the brink and back many times before allowing you to release in orgasm. Take your lover to the brink and back again with breast play, and tease abundantly before taking her breasts fully into your mouth.

➔ *Top Ten Titillating Tips*

1. Start gently, go slow, and don't treat the region above the waist like a chore, like a stepping-stone to the real deal. Sex is not all about intercourse.
2. Be respectful. Don't presume to help yourself to a handful without invitation. In other words, don't just plunge your hands under her shirt, then beneath her bra, and start squeezing. *Tease* and *trace* are two key words for breast play.
3. Pay attention to body language; don't just do it by the book. Be creative, and go beyond a sloppy squeeze. Breast play is not like shaking hands. Ask her what she likes. Ask her to show you how she would like to be touched.
4. Give her emotional strokes, not just physical strokes. Tell her how beautiful her breasts are, Romeo. Nestle your head in them and appreciate them, whatever their size.
5. Create drama and suspense. Be a tease, and don't rush to conclusion. Move from a breast to her neck, then back to her lips, then back down to her other breast. Or kiss down

to her belly button or thereabouts, then back up to her other breast.

6. Involve all her senses. Breasts go with so many things: ice, honey, mangoes, champagne, scented massage oil . . .

7. Never fall into a pattern of predictability; dazzle her with your inventiveness. Use the different strokes covered in the "Massage" section of the next chapter on her chest. Kiss your way in concentric circles to her nipple, then do a surprise attack on it—no warning, no prisoners—stealing away her breath.

8. Don't be afraid to get kinky or rough if that's what she likes. Pinch and pull her nipple or give it a loving spanking with the tongue tip of a belt. You can also use clamps or other toys, like a vibrator, on her breasts.

9. If you move into other activities, don't forget the breasts. Keep them as active players in the sex dance. Remember, you're making love to her entire body, mind, and spirit. A lot of women love the simultaneous stimulation of breasts and genitals. So while your mouth is wrapped around her love box, stroke her breasts with your magic fingers!

10. At the end of a lovemaking session, give her breasts a final caress.

When it comes to breasts and nipples, experiment with movements subtle and unpredictable, varying both speed and style, confusing her with nibbling, lapping, tiny nips, and the occasional deep-throating of the entire breast into your hot mouth, where it can be bathed lovingly with tongue strokes.

☀ *Masturbation: Not So-lo!*

Each woman has different needs for how she likes to be touched. We've already discussed the importance of communicating our wants and desires. Now understand that words don't always convey what a demonstration can. Masturbation as part of sex is a hot way to enjoy each other's bodies and learn firsthand what your partner likes.

> *Masturbating with partners is one of my favorite things. It is hot because I know I'll get off, and I learn a lot from my partner's technique about how to please her.*
> —Carrie, 25, San Francisco

> *I would not masturbate for a lover, because I think the point of a lover is to not have to masturbate.*
> —Judy, 20, Memphis, Tennessee

Masturbation is not a self-indulgent waste of time. It is not reserved solely for folks without current sexual partners, for filling the gaps when the nookie supply is low. It can be an important means of self-discovery and self-expression for you and your lover.

Encouraging Her to Learn Her Body

Masturbation is one area of sex where men seem to be a little more active than women—or at least they're more out about it. Most lesbians tend to be comfortable with it because they're used to touching pussy and they enjoy it! And many straight women also have a healthy masturbation appetite.

But there is a faction of heterosexual women who have more hangups about touching their genitals. So uncomfortable are they that they would never consider using a diaphragm or cervical cap as a method of birth control because either would require them to touch their vulva when inserting them.

If you have a partner who doesn't have orgasms, it's probably because she doesn't know how, not because she can't. The best way for her to learn how to come—and to teach you how to help her do so—is to masturbate. This allows her to explore her body and touch herself in various ways to see what feels good to her. If she has internalized negative messages, she may feel weird about masturbating or even be adamant about not doing it. This is where your encouragement and support can be helpful.

Be a Self-loving Coach

She likes it when I move her own hand in between her legs.
—John, 35, Pasadena, California

She may not feel comfortable doing it by herself—but she may do it with you as part of sex. Ask her to show you how she likes to be touched. If she is not having orgasms with you, explain to her how much it would help to be able to watch her bring herself to orgasm. Tell her you'll be right there and will do whatever she wants to aid in the process. That might include sucking her breasts, caressing her body, kissing her, telling her a hot story, or all of the above. Be a great coach.

If she's still being hesitant about it, you might have to get more active. Choose a time when she is relaxed and you are engaged in some kissing, body-rubbing, or other turn-ons. Wait for an appropriate opportunity, then gently take her hand and put it on her pussy. Keep your hand on top of hers and stay with her. If her hand sits there stiff and scared like a deer caught in the headlights, continue, in your gentle fashion, moving her hand with yours to help her get into the groove. Like a cat nudging its head into you so you'll pet him, nudge her to pet herself. If she really doesn't feel comfortable, don't force anything.

In the best-case scenario, she'll get into it so much that she won't even notice when you take your hand away and she'll continue stimulating herself to orgasm. Pay close attention so you can do a repeat performance later on.

And if all this hard work doesn't do the trick, buy her a vibrator and be her vibrator coach!

I love it when she pleasures herself and enjoys watching me pleasure myself. It's a high form of intimacy.
—Larry, 61, a small town in Tennessee

> *I masturbate with and for my partners because I think it brings about a certain intimacy level that is important in a relationship. Also, it generally involves a certain amount of trust, and that is also important.*
>
> —Jasmine, 18, Charleston, South Carolina

Give Her Some Bath Love

Water can be a great sex toy. One popular method of masturbation for many women is to run bathwater over the vulva. Many girls learn to masturbate as children in this innocent way. That childhood association can even be a turn-on for some.

If you want to give her a special treat, set everything up for a bath, minus the water. Light the candles, sprinkle the rose petals, light the incense, and place a bath pillow on the tub floor near the faucet so she doesn't get a bruised tailbone. If you don't have one, a towel will work; it will just be sopping wet when you're through. Then bring her in, turn on the water, and have her adjust it to a comfortable temperature. Pussies usually won't want the water as steamy as a sore body would—we don't want any scalded labia!

Have her sit on the pillow and scoot her bottom up under the faucet so the water is running over her vulva. You can sit behind her so she can lean on you or put her head in your lap with her legs hiked up on the wall and her pussy directly under the water's flow. You'll have a great angle from which to watch her and help her out by caressing her breasts, body, or head. Talk to her, encourage her, tell her how lovely she looks. Watch the movement of her body as the water cleanses and satisfies her clit. Just sit back and appreciate her pleasure as you fill the bath. Many women can reach a yummy, comforting orgasm this way.

> *I like watching how she touches herself, and just seeing her writhe and feel good. You don't get to enjoy observing the lovely shape and nuance of a woman's body when you are constantly in her face.*   —Brian, 30, New York

Show 'n' Tell and Genital Massage for Partners

Remember first-grade show 'n' tell? Remember how fun it was to bring something you cared about to class for the opportunity to share it with all your friends? Remember all the interesting stuff your classmates brought in?

Well, let's hearken back to those days with a special kind of show 'n' tell. You remember this one, when you and the girl down the block got together and one of you eagerly said, "I'll show you mine if you show me yours."

This is a fabulous way to get back to your child self and learn a lot about your partner in the process. If you want, this is another excellent way to start a mutual masturbation session. All you need is a cozy place, a little stand-up mirror, and plenty of time and attention.

Take turns showing each other your genitals. You can sit facing each other, or side by side using a mirror. A mirror is helpful, so you both can see yourselves as you describe the various parts of your genitals and why you like them. You can go through the parts and talk about what feels good to them. It's like drawing a little map of your pleasure for your lover.

After you take turns looking at each other and asking questions, you can move into some genital self-massage. This is different from masturbating, although it might be arousing. You are not working toward a goal or working for orgasm. You are massaging for the sake of massage, to wake up your nerves, release tension you might be holding, and appreciate your genitals.

Both of you should be very thorough. Use a bit of massage oil, and give every bit of your genitals some attention. She can stroke and pull her outer lips, pinch and pull the inner lips, work down her shaft, circle around her vaginal opening, stroke around the entire perimeter of the vulva, massage the perineum and the anus. She can also put a finger inside her vagina and/or anus and massage around the walls of each. We discuss genital massage in more detail in the following chapter.

Guys, don't think of it as masturbation. Give yourself a real genital massage. Work all the places that usually don't get touched. You can knead your testicles and the whole length of your penis. Put the fingers of both hands on either side of your shaft and work in short strokes from the base to the tip. Then work on your perineum and the outside of your anus. If you are comfortable with it, insert your finger or thumb into your anus and massage the inside.

Oil will help your strokes, but don't overdo it or it gets too slick. After your self-massages, you can move into mutual masturbation if you want. If any of this leads to any activities that will require latex, remember to wash off the oil first so your latex stays intact.

Keep Your Hands on Yourself

> *I think it's a terrific turn-on to masturbate in front of a lover or to watch a man masturbate. Educational, too. It's one way to have safe sex at the beginning of a relationship before the trust level is very high. Yay for masturbation!*
> —Jeannie, 52, Tampa, Florida

> *It's such a cool thing to watch someone take themselves to orgasm. It makes me feel like a voyeur and very trusted.*
> —Suzanne, 29, New York

Mutual masturbation is one of the hottest ways to get to know your partner and how she likes to be touched, as well as to teach her what you like. For many people it does require a certain level of trust, because it is such an intimate thing to share with someone. What better way is there to learn about each other and get a big ol' turn-on at the same time 'cause you get to watch? Relax. All roads do not have to lead to intercourse, so take a new road. As a matter of fact, mutual masturbation is its own form of intercourse. So get in touch with your inner voyeur, and pull up a front-row seat for the best interactive show you could dream of.

Creating a Master-Date

Start by creating an environment that appeals to both of you. You might take that candlelit bath together, washing each other and gracing bodies with kisses. It will be an entire night of pampering yourselves. But before moving into the bathroom for that sweet dip in the tub, set up the room you will retire to after the bath with some burning incense and romantic lighting. (Just don't leave candles burning while you're gone—fire hazard!) It keeps the flow of the evening consistent when the mood you've created is maintained everywhere. Nobody wants to exit the warm, sweet, candlelit bathroom and enter a bedroom with harsh, bright lights. Make sure the space is ready.

You can have the whole masturbation session in the bath if you want to, although water can impede manual stimulation depending on how you do it. Water isn't a great lubricant. Otherwise, just spend time washing each other, relaxing, and enjoying the water. When you're ready to get out, you will enter a warm, good-smellin' parlor o' mutual pleasure.

You set the rules together. Your rule could be "There are no rules." But if you aren't that disciplined, let us suggest a few:

1. Keep your hands on your own genitals! No exceptions!
2. Keep your mouths and genitals to yourself.
3. Encouraging or sensuous talk is allowed. This is to be a mutually supportive activity.
4. Both partners will masturbate manually to orgasm, however long it takes.

You can use some or all of these and add others. You can do whatever you want later, but right now it's just the two of you, your bodies and your self-pleasure.

Put on some music you both like if you want, or do it in silence so all you hear is each other. We suggest rule number 4 because part of the mission is to learn how you each like to be stimulated so you can incorporate what you learn in future sexual encounters. But, no pressure!

Sit so you are both comfortable and can see each other. It's important to face each other, so you can really take in the eroticism of each other's bodies and arousal. You can make contact with your feet or legs. Be playful, have fun with it, and enjoy watching your partner. Be the voyeur you always wanted to be. Act out a fantasy if you want. You can set up whatever situation you like, as long as you masturbate together. Make it a peep show and pretend there is a glass partition between you. However you do it, this will be an illuminating date that you and your partner will not soon forget. You'll both reap the benefits as you learn to better pleasure each other and develop a stronger intimate bond. One woman shared the following story, which shows how you can use communication for erotic play.

A Lesson on Erotic Dates

One of the hottest things a lover ever did to me happened on our first date. She was a butch top, and I was really attracted to her sexual confidence and knew she'd take me somewhere new. That excited me a whole lot, and I was ready to get down and go wherever she might take me.

Finally, the date. After dinner, she suggested we go back to my place. We did, and after talking and listening to music for a long while, she asked me to put on some sexy music I liked and to light some candles. I immediately complied, wondering what she was up to.

Next, she had me strip down, one article of clothing at a time. She first asked me to remove my shirt, then my belt, then my pants, and after each article came off, she took a moment to appreciate what was revealed. For the exhibitionist in me this was totally hot, and I complied willingly. She asked me to lie down next to her, and what followed was the most thorough investigation of my body's pleasure spots anyone had ever taken the time for. And this was only our first date!

Starting with my neck and face, she touched me and kissed me in every nook and cranny, in every different way, asking with each bit how much I liked it. She gave me a pleasure scale of 1 to 10, 10 being most pleasurable, as a mode of response.

"Do you like to have your neck kissed, like this?" she'd ask, giving my neck sweet kisses.

"Ooh, 7½!"

"What about having your neck bitten, like this?" she said, nibbling on my neck.

"Mmmm, 9½!"

"Do you like your breasts to be licked like this?"

"Umm, 7."

"Pulled, like this?"

"Oh, that's a 9!"

She worked down my arms, wrists, hands, breasts, torso, tummy, thighs, all the way down my legs to my toes and the bottoms of my feet, back up my body, over my butt, every inch of my back and head. She didn't miss a spot.

Then she stopped. I wanted to kiss her, but she wouldn't let me. Tease. Mind you, she was still fully clothed. Then this was the clincher. She asked me to show her how I masturbate.

"I usually use a vibrator," I said.

"Okay, so get it out and show me."

With a sly smile, I reached under my bed and produced my vibrator. She didn't blink an eye. I leaned back and began to masturbate.

"Oh, and don't forget to ask permission to come," she said matter-of-factly.

"Excuse me?" I said.

"You need to ask permission. When you're ready to come, let me know."

I'd never had to ask permission. But I was well-behaved and enjoyed the ride, with no expectations for where it would go. It was obvious who was in charge, and that was just fine with me. She knew I was attracted to her confidence and her role as a top. I masturbated for her, and she made me stop three or four times before I could come. She finally allowed me to come, nuzzling her ear up next to my face so she could listen close. I had a huge orgasm, a total euphoric release.

It was one of the most sensuous, erotic experiences of my life. What made it so amazing was all her attention to details, the time she took to introduce herself to my body and find out everything she could about what it likes and doesn't like, learning from the get-go how to touch me. I was the one eager to get down and dirty with her, but she held me off, asserting her power as a top, and I was incredibly grateful. I learned a lot about her that night as well, and she ended up being one of the most amazing lovers of my life, certainly the one I grew the most with sexually.

If people made a habit of taking that kind of time to get to know their lovers, to explore their bodies, to listen to them, to watch them pleasure themselves, and to simply enjoy them without being focused on a goal or on themselves, sex would reach totally new realms of mutual pleasure. This is not to say she didn't have any goals in mind. But her goals were to get to know me and my body and my desire. That was the beginning of one passionate and very sensual relationship.

This is one example of how you can get to know a partner under the right conditions. Obviously, a lot of comfort is needed for something like that, and it may not be the same for you. Come up with your own ideas and style for acquainting yourself with your lovers. We've given you a few ideas—embellish them, and do it your way. Listen, learn, and incorporate! What could make sex better? If you know her well, you'll do her well!

Sapphic
Arts

☀️ Massage

Physical touch is not only powerful; it's necessary for our well-being. We know that when people do not get enough touch as infants and children, their growth is stunted, sometimes dramatically. We all need loving, caring touch. It heals us to have body and energetic contact with another human being. A simple hug has the power to cure our doldrums.

> *Massage is so sensuous. It makes me feel like he loves my body for what it is, not just for sex.*
> —Michelle, 30, Sherman Oaks, California

> *My girlfriend and I love to exchange massage. We use candles, incense, and music to create a relaxing space. It helps us both reduce stress and it feels good to service her body in such an intimate way.* —Nicky, 25, Montreal

A loving massage of our entire body will leave us warm, relaxed, loved, and rejuvenated. If you have yet to incorporate massage into your intimate relationships, there is no better time than the present to give it a whirl.

Hands On

In many lesbian relationships massage is a primary player. Massage is a form of sensuous touch that can be sexual or non-sexual. It's a great way of tuning in and connecting to your partner. It's also a good way to build trust for allowing others to touch our body in an intimate way. And everyone loves a good backrub.

Sometimes lovers don't give a good backrub because they're lazy. And sometimes it's kind of like busting moves out on the dance floor—they're a little shy and unsure of their strokes because they don't want to be considered a loser in the backrub department, going down with the unimpressive nickname "Bad Hands."

> *Massage is loving touch. Loving touch is basic to being a lover. For us, massage can happen whenever one of us needs it or wants it, or when one of us really wants to give one, which can be part of the dance of foreplay, too. She likes having her feet massaged, and I like doing it. When a woman gives you her feet, she is inviting intimacy.*
> —Lee, 54, Northbrook, Illinois

This chapter will give some basic moves so you never have to say no because you feel inadequate. One of the most important parts of being a good lover is giving. Don't be lazy. The power of touch is one of the greatest healers and stress relievers on the planet, better than any over-the-counter or prescription drug.

Erotic and Sensual

A sensual massage is about relaxing, and relieving stress and tension in the body. It's about health and wellness.

☼ Honey, Come Closer

Massage can be very erotic, arousing, healing, and exciting. Erotic massage can include the genitals but doesn't have to. This does not mean erotic massage has to end in sexual play, but it very well might include stimulation that leads to heightened states of sexual pleasure and orgasm. It can open up the sexual center and build trust and familiarity, making sex more enjoyable.

Through your touch and her feedback, you'll discover which strokes your partner likes, where she holds tension, how much pressure she prefers, and what parts of her body need a little extra attention. This body communication can open up a similar communication in your sexual relationship, and in the relationship in general. It's a safe and emotionally connected way to relate to each other's body, mind, and spirit. Plus, it feels great!

Creating the Ritual

> *I think the nicest thing a partner can do for you is to massage your body. Not only does it create intimacy between the two of you, but you become more intimate with yourself. They're allowing you to feel every part of yourself too, to be awakened.* —Claudia, 22, New Rochelle, New York

It's key to have a warm, cozy environment. Your lover's body temperature will drop during a massage. If she's cold, her body will tense up, and that will counteract some benefits of the massage. It's a good idea to have extra towels to keep the areas you just worked on warm and a couple of extra pillows for your lover's head or for under her knees when she's on her back. Relaxing music, candles, and soft light make for a safe, inviting environment.

Oils

Massage oil makes for effective, friction-free strokes. You can buy premixed scented oils or use a nice organic almond or sunflower oil. Make sure your hands are warm before your first touch. If they aren't, rub them together to warm them, then rub the oil between your hands to warm it up. You can even warm the oil in a coffee mug of hot water before you use it. Just put the whole bottle in the cup for a few minutes and that should do the trick.

Do It 'Cause You Wanna

Give your lover a massage without expecting one in return. She can return the favor another day.

Give it for the sake of giving. Your reward will be the joy you get from loving her body in this way.

> ### ː♡ː Honey, Come Closer
>
> The last thing someone should feel obligated to do after a nice, yummy, relaxing massage is get up and use all those freshly relaxed muscles to work on somebody else! That defeats the purpose. Let the massage be a gift.

First Contact

When you start the massage, you want to make sure your energy is centered. Take some deep breaths, feel your feet connected to the floor, and let any mental distractions go. Like good sex, a good massage requires you to be fully present. This is a chance for you to let some of your own stress go and focus on your partner instead of yourself. Take a few minutes to look at her body before you even touch her. Really focus on it, look at its shape, and notice any obvious tense spots.

The first touch should be a simple laying of hands on your lover's body. Start with her lower back, then move up her spine, applying a little more pressure as you go, telling her to breathe and release. These first moments are about connecting with her, making her feel safe, and tuning in to her body.

The Massage Path

When you give a massage, you normally work one area at a time, then work into others. You might start with her neck and back, move down the back of her legs, then have her turn over and work the front of her torso, the front of her legs, and her arms. Don't forget her hands and feet! In each of these areas you can get more specific, zeroing in on the areas where she really needs it, then finishing the area with broad general strokes. It's best to keep talking to a minimum. Do the massage silently or with soothing music so she can just lie back and relax.

Final Touches

It's good to end the massage with some long, gentle strokes that connect all the areas, then lightly brush the body off with feather strokes. If your lover is on her back, place one hand on her forehead and the other just above her pubic bone and sit peacefully for a minute to connect the energy. Then slowly raise your hands and glide them slowly over her body just above the surface of her skin without touching it. Tell her to open her eyes when she's ready. If she is on her stomach, you can do the same sequence by placing your hands on the small of her back and the back of her neck. Then you can give her some private time or lie down beside her and cuddle.

☼♡☼ Honey, Come Closer

It's a great idea to go get a massage for yourself if you've never had one. You can learn more from a trained professional than we could possibly explain here about how to touch a lover's body. You will give better massages too, since you will know what different strokes feel like to the receiver.

Different Strokes

Long Strokes

The following two strokes are designed to run the length of your partner's body, either from her butt to the top of her shoulders or from the ankle to the butt. If your partner is on her back, you can use these strokes from her shoulders, across her breasts to the bottom of her abdomen as well. Don't be shy about touching her butt with these strokes. No pressure should ever be applied to the sensitive joints—use light touches around knees, elbows, wrists, and ankles.

Flat Hands. The stroke most of us intuitively use when rubbing someone's back is perfect for opening a massage treatment. With relaxed flat hands, apply pressure on the forward stroke and lighten it on the return. The heel of your hand does most of the work. It's a great stroke for the back because of the large surface area. You place your hands at the top of your lover's butt on either side of the spine, then stroke upward toward her shoulders, returning by circling to the outside. This relaxes her and prepares her for deeper strokes.

Cupped Hands. This stroke is great for the back of the legs. The calves are pretty sensitive because many people carry tension there. Starting just above the ankle, place your hands next to each other, thumbs touching, fingers pointing in the same direction. Cup your hands to match the contour of her legs. Gently stroke up the leg to the butt. Follow the same technique as with flat hands, with pressure on the forward movement and a light touch on the return. This mode of pressure helps carry waste products to the lymph glands for elimination.

Squeezing

Squeezing techniques work well on the legs, butt, and shoulders. Squeezing and wringing will help release tension and relax the muscles. They help break up those knots caused by stress, emotional upset, or other imbalances that manifest in our bodies. They need some kneading out, or they just stay lodged there, causing pain and discomfort.

Cup and Squeeze. Anchoring one of your lover's legs at the ankle with one hand, use the other hand to work your way up the outside of the leg as you squeeze, slightly rotating the wrist upward as you move toward the butt. Then switch hands, repeat the motion on the inside of the leg, and move on to the other leg.

Going Both Ways. This is another treat for the legs. Place your hands just below her buttock, wrists touching, with the fingers of one hand pointing down the inside of her leg and the others pointing down the outside. Pressing with the heels of your hands, push out to each side of the leg, then bring your hands back together. Use this motion all the way down the leg, moving a hand's width at a time, then repeat with the other leg.

Two-Handed Cross. This is a great stroke for the large muscles of the butt. Lay both hands on one butt cheek, thumbs side by side, and move the heel of your hands back-and-forth across the butt. Then do her other cheek for balance. You can also use this stroke to work up and down the leg.

Wringing. Using both hands, keeping an inch or two of distance between them, wring your lover's arm or leg as if you are wringing a towel, moving up or down the length of the muscles. Be sure to check in with her to see how much pressure she is comfortable with.

Kneading. It helps to lean your body weight into this stroke—good for any muscle area—before you start the motion. Firmly grasp the muscle between your thumb and fingers and squeeze, rhythmically kneading your lover's flesh. Slow, deep strokes will help release tension and toxins. Faster strokes will increase stimulation, energizing the body. You can knead an entire muscle area or focus on a particular spot.

Knuckles

Knuckles are useful for hard-to-get places, like tie-in points between muscles or underneath the shoulder blade. They are also good for more specific work, like the upper chest, the back of the neck, and the shoulders, and feel great on the bottoms of the feet.

Under the Knuckle. You can use one or two knuckles in circular motion to do deep pressure-point work and ease areas of tension. Those tension knots we described earlier are often pressure points that are good to work out. Or you can make a fist and use your knuckles in a gliding motion. This is effective in fleshy areas like the back of the legs and the butt.

Percussion

Percussive movements are good for breaking up toxic and fatty deposits and waking up an area in general. Be careful, though, to stay away from any traumatized or bony areas. Percussion is safe for the butt and the thighs. It is also effective for the trapezius, that muscle on your back, just above the shoulders and behind the neck, where a lot of people hold tension. The key to any good percussion technique is relaxed hands and wrists and a solid, steady rhythm.

Pounding, Tapping, and Chopping. These three techniques are similar. The main differences are hand positions. With all of them, you rapidly and continually drum down on the skin. Pounding is done with a loosely closed fist, chopping with an open hand like a karate chop. Tapping is very light percussion done with the fingertips—good for a gentle wake-up or for sensitive and bony areas, and also great for the scalp.

> *Massage has taught me so much about my lover's body. I know where she holds her tension and which places turn her on.*   —Kerri, 27, Madison, Wisconsin

Other Techniques

Circles. Use your fingertips to work deeply into an area by moving in a slow, tight circular motion.

Pinches and Pulls. For this little technique, pinch a piece of skin lightly, pulling up and letting go. Generously working an area with repetitive love pinches will ease the muscles and break up tension deposits.

Feathers. Long, soft feather strokes make a good finisher. Run your fingertips lightly down your partner's entire body, extending all the way to the end of the limbs, gradually lightening the contact with each stroke until you are just gliding slightly above the skin. If you have some large ostrich feathers (if nothing else, some cat toys are made out of them), stroking the skin with them is a sweet, gentle way to finish as well.

The Genitals

When you become interested in another person sexually, the sensation of attraction can be felt in the genital region. Your mind and even your heart may be engaged, but you probably feel it first and best in your groin. So it should come as no surprise that each sexual rejection, abandonment, or disappointment may become lodged in your genital area. Our genitals have pressure points and hold tension like any other part of the body. Layer upon layer of painful brushoffs, letdowns, or unsatisfying sex can create energy blocks that can be removed or relieved through genital massage.

The problem with most massages is that they bypass crucial parts of the body like the breasts, buttocks, and genitals because those areas are "sexual." Yep, they're sexual, but they need massage and therapeutic touch as much as any other part of the body. We are accustomed to stimulating, masturbating, or playing with our genitals, but how often do they get a loving massage for massage's sake, instead of with the goal of sexual excitement?

If you are massaging a lover you are comfortable with, don't leave out her genitals. Be gentle and massage her vulva as you would the other parts of her body. You are not massaging to sexually arouse her, although if you do it well, some arousal might be unavoidable. Massage her vulva to release the tension she may be carrying there. If you relax her genitals, they will flower and open, and if you both have the energy when you are finished, it could be the best warm-up for a lovemaking session. If either one of you doesn't have the energy or isn't in the mood, just cuddle up and drift off to sleep.

Genital Massage

Wash your hands thoroughly (get under those fingernails!), pour some warmed oil into them. Start by putting one hand on her vulva and the other on her heart for a moment. Then begin to massage her from the belly to the pubic mound and upper thighs. Spend time making slow, firm circles around the mons and the outer lips. A pinching technique will work well for her labia. Gently pinch and rub the sensitive outer and inner labia between your thumbs and index fingers. Do both sides simultaneously, taking your time and working all the way up and down the length of each lip.

Run your thumbs along the sides of the clitoral shaft, all the way down the crease of her inner lips. Take a thumb and gently rub in a circular motion just inside the vestibule—just be careful not to irritate her urethra. Slowly, methodically, and deliberately, circle with both thumb tips until every centimeter of the labia is massaged.

Once the outer vulva is sufficiently massaged, slip an index finger into the vagina. Just barely inside the entrance, apply pressure in a small circular motion around the inner edges. Then work your way around the inside like a clock, stopping at each position, one through twelve, and massage in a small circular motion. Be gentle. After each trip around the clock, move your finger in deeper. When you are finished, cup your hand over her vulva for a minute or two. You will probably feel her heart beating, because the blood will be flowing in her genitals.

Be aware that this can be a powerful emotional experience. Emotional body blows, sexual assaults, and car wrecks can get recorded there. This massage can open the area up, causing an emotional flood of tears. Such a release will ultimately make your lover more trusting and responsive.

➡ *Good Reasons to Get Into Massage*

1. It's a ritual that makes you spend quality, sensual time together, appreciating your lover's body without expecting something in return.
2. It's fun and it feels great and it's cheaper than renting porn.
3. It's process oriented instead of goal oriented.
4. It's a form of safer sex.

5. It helps you learn to communicate physically.
6. You learn a lot about your lover's body, how she likes to be touched and her hot spots.

Massage is a safe way to connect with your lover physically, erotically, and emotionally. Make it part of your life.

☀ *Finger Love: Becoming a Digital Master*

You know why women love musicians? Because musicians are creative, and they make their living with their mouth and hands. Major turn-on! It would be a great help if you start thinking about your hands as the delicate and precise tools of a piano player, guitarist, or sculptor. Don't underestimate the power of your hands to leave your partner gleefully satisfied.

♡ Honey, Come Closer

A steady hand is worth a thousand orgasms. Your hands are adaptable tools of pleasure. Just let the idea of your hands' being highly sensitive and coordinated love tools work on you, and you're on your way to becoming a virtuoso.

It's in Your Hands

Susie Bright, lesbian sexpert extraordinaire, was the sex consultant for the hot lesbian flick *Bound*, featuring Gina Gershon and Jennifer Tilly. What a job! Gina played the sexy, butch handywoman, and Susie's advice to her and to the director was that for a believable lesbian portrayal, it was all in her hands. Be assured, many a woman will notice your hands, wondering what they will feel like on her skin, how they will touch her, if they will arouse her. Women often have softer hands than many men. The lesbian women we surveyed spoke of that as a definite plus in having women as sexual partners. Women have softer skin, and soft skin often likes to be touched and graced with soft hands. Some women, though, like a nice pair of rugged hands. The details vary, but be assured, your hands will be very important.

> *Usually right before I orgasm, if they are in reach, I grab my partner's hands to squeeze in mine. It makes me feel safe and connected.* —Jamila, 34, Philadelphia

Too many men never use their hands to really explore their partners' bodies. They kiss and go right for her pants, perhaps with a short detour at her breasts. If you have participated in this kind of unbecoming behavior, leave it in the past! She wants her whole body to be touched and awakened, the nerve endings that extend along and beyond her whole spine to be ignited with touch. Spend time touching her, stroking her, massaging her, loving her entire body. Do not miss an inch. A man with good hands is a rare jewel she won't easily let go of, or forget.

> *Always be aware of where your hands are, no matter what you're doing. Whether they are active or not, use them to connect to your partner. I had a lover who always wrapped my arms and hands under and around her spread thighs when I would go down on her. It made her feel embraced and safe.* —Tiffany, 31, Boston

The first thing you need to do is look at your hands in a new way—not for throwing a football, not for using power tools (well, we take that back), not for flipping channels, but as versatile tools of love. Most guys use their fingers like they use their penis. Don't be silly. You castrate the power of your hands when you do that!

Finger Love 101

Finger sex is not about thrusting a stiff index finger in and out of your lover's pussy (though thrusting is one of the many things your fingers can do). Don't feel bad if that's the way you've been doing it. You probably were never taught this fine art by a patient and explicit teacher. And maybe your partner doesn't know any better either. So don't think of it as finger fucking, think of it as finger love. In your fingers, you have ten sweet partner pleasers.

Your fingers are potentially very dexterous and nimble, but too often in sex they're used as if they were paws. You need to learn how to relax your hands, apply subtle degrees of pressure, and become adept at gradual and specific motions.

Just realizing that your fingers have this potential and applying it when you're making love will automatically make for a big improvement. Your mind is incredibly powerful when properly directed. You'll probably find a light, delicate touch the most difficult and fatiguing to sustain, but when dealing with the softness of women's bodies and the often extreme sensitivity of the clitoris, it'll be necessary to use your finger stamina. So strengthen them if necessary.

Digitizing Her Vulva

Your hands can touch your partner's center of pleasure, her clitoris, in the focused, controlled, and specific way that most clits need. It can feel really good to your partner if you rub your hard cock all over her vulva and clit, but for sustained clitoral stimulation, you've got to use your hands or other implements, like a vibrator or a tongue.

Tease Her!

When beginning manual stimulation, don't just go straight for the clit. Make her really want it. Work your way slowly to the clitoris. Start by sensitizing the area around her vulva, including the inner thighs and the belly. Stroke softly, tease, kiss, invite goose bumps. Then stroke her whole pubic area and outer lips with a feather-light touch. Build up painfully slow. Make her want more, spreading her legs, her pelvis rising toward you, eager for more pressure. When she's ready, make her wait just a little longer.

> *Most men I've been with go right for my clit. The clit has gotten so much hype as this magic button, men think all they have to do is make a beeline to it and I'm going to have an orgasm or want to immediately have sex.*
>
> —Kimberly, 34, Cleveland

Be Gentle

As a man you're probably used to delivering a firmer touch. After all, that's the way you learned to shake hands, or it might be the way you masturbate. Men are more physical with their little soldier. The penis can take it—it doesn't mind a little dick whacking.

The clitoris is more sensitive. If you compare its size to that of the penis, it makes sense: Women have more nerve endings clustered in their clitoris (a much smaller space) than men have in their penis. Like we said, finger finesse and some light, delicate touching will be what many women prefer, at least at first. You don't want to get too rough with a clit unless you are specifically invited to do so.

> *My boyfriend masturbated for me, and I was surprised at how forceful he was with himself. Especially as he reached orgasm. He started going really fast and hard. It looked like he was hurting himself.* —Carolyn, 27, Fresno, California

Don't assume that she likes to be rubbed like you do. It is best, with the clitoris, to start out with soft and gentle touching until you are directed otherwise. And when you are directed, be a good actor and make the adjustment in the scene.

Positioning

For lasting finger love, you want to find a comfortable position. The most awkward position is sitting between her legs facing her. It's hard to duplicate what she likes from this angle, and it puts a lot of pressure on your wrists. That doesn't mean this position is a no-no. Maybe she comes like a volcano when you stimulate her from there.

From a side-by-side position, you can rest your wrist on her pubic area with your fingers dropped down over her vulva to stimulate it. You can also reach inside her from this position. Or you can sit behind her while she leans back against you, wrapped between your legs—you can kiss her neck, caress her breast, or pinch her nipples with your free hand, and she'll feel soft and warm leaning into you.

⚡♡⚡ Honey, Come Closer

Rule number one in finger love: Never touch a dry clit or enter a dry vagina with a dry finger. Just as most men use some kind of lubricant when they masturbate for a smoother glide, women need it too.

Lubricants

Touching a dry clit creates friction that can be uncomfortable or annoying at best and downright painful at worst. Either get some pussy juice up on the clit, lick your fingers, or use some artificial lubricant. Some women may need only a little bit, while others will like copious lubrication. If you put too much, she may not get enough friction, so you want to check in with her about that. Use artificial lubricant if her own juice isn't enough. If you can get it from her pussy, do it. One woman said she found it offensive if a partner used artificial lubricant without first checking and trying to get it from her pussy naturally. We've all got preferences. You want to have lube on hand, but reserve it for when au naturel doesn't cut the mustard. If you want to be safer and avoid any fluid exchange via your mouth, have her salivate on your fingers by sucking on them. Be aware that saliva often dries up quickly, and so does her pussy juice if it's not abundant.

Always keep your fingers and her clit moist and slick. Don't assume that lubricating them once will do the job. You have to keep refueling. Sometimes artificial lube, depending on the type, will last longer and won't dry up. Some types do dry quickly. You can remedy this by keeping some water by the bedside so you can wet your fingers now and then. When you add a little water, the lube will slick right back up for more bang for your buck. If you are planning to go down on her, the artificial lube might not taste so good, and might take away from the pleasure of the act, unless you got one of the flavored varieties. So keep that in mind.

Finger Fucking

Now that she's warmed up and maybe even had an orgasm, you can bring a little penetration into the mix. But don't forget all you've learned. Thrusting a dry finger into a dry pussy is not a fun activity for most women. The more you arouse the rest of her body, kiss her, and stimulate her clitoris, the juicier her pussy will get and the more fun it will be when something enters it. Don't be too eager now.

> *I've got to be wet for a finger to feel good. If a lover tries to insert and finds it's dry, then don't go there. Having a finger inside me won't make me wet. It will be unpleasant.*
> —Carol, 22, Memphis, Tennessee

Your fingers have distinct advantages for sexing her up on the inside. They can reach all the nooks and crannies of her vagina that bring her pleasure. Have them hang out around the opening at first and choose the perfect moment, after lots of teasing, to enter her.

Keep in mind that the outer third of the vagina has the most nerve endings. You don't necessarily need to go deep. Don't stick your finger in all at once! Start with the tip. Once inside, swirl your fingertip around the rim. Then slowly work your finger in a little farther and continue to explore. Some women get off on cervical stimulation. Depending on the length of your fingers and the depth of her vagina, you might be able to reach back and touch her cervix.

Some women like some in-and-out thrusting. Others prefer that you insert one or two fingers, keep them in, and move them around on the inside. Some like you to just keep them still, because they like the feeling of having something in their vagina. Many women prefer a combination of styles.

> *I like it when he starts out with one finger until I'm relaxed, then adds a second. But he needs to take his time on the second, working his way slowly in. Not just jamming two in because he's already had one in.*
>
> —Denise, 29, Phoenix

> *I like a finger in there, but please don't dig for China.*
>
> —Pam, 33, Houston

The best part about using your finger(s) inside her pussy is that you are able to really feel what goes on inside her as her arousal builds and as she comes to orgasm. This can be just as much of a turn-on for you as it is for her. Plus, you can more easily determine which things turn her on most. Be conscious of the subtle shifts and changes that occur when you are inside of her. She might find it really hot if you whisper in her ear what you are feeling, what is happening in her body, and what you like about it. This shows you are paying attention, and she might really like hearing your voice or hearing you talk dirty. It will also help her learn. Because of the extensive system of nerves, muscles, and blood flow in their pelvises, women can't always feel exactly where certain sensations are coming from. When you give her specifics, she will understand the mechanisms in her own body better. So get into it and give it to her with poetry!

The G-Spot

Your fingers have the best chance of stimulating her urethral sponge (G-spot), discussed earlier in the "How Women Work" chapter. It's on the top or front wall of her vagina, usually just inside, remember? Curling your finger toward the front wall or pressing against it as you thrust in and out should stimulate it. Insert one or two fingers and do the come-here motion. Some women get incredibly aroused by this. But it's important to know that many women won't like it at all, so if it doesn't work for her, focus your attention elsewhere.

> ### ♡ Honey, Come Closer
>
> While you stimulate her G-spot, you might also want to stimulate her clitoris with your thumb, your other hand, or your mouth. Many women love the combination of G-spot and clitoral stimulation. As her arousal builds, you should feel her sponge enlarge and protrude more as it engorges with blood.

Also, if you turn your finger toward her backside, you can stimulate her perineal sponge.

Remember that while many women love to have their G-spots played with, there are many others who will get nothing out of it and might actually find it annoying. There is nothing wrong with that. Just focus your attention elsewhere.

Digital Strokes

There are a hundred ways to manually stimulate her pussy. The following are a few variations you can play with. Have fun!

- Simply use the pads of your fingers over the top half of the vulva. Apply some pressure. Use multiple fingers, and you will cover more terrain; you can get the whole shaft, glans, and part of the lips this way.

- Lay your whole hand over the vulva and use it to stimulate her in a motion she likes. Gripping the outer lips and clitoral shaft and moving in a circular motion will stimulate most of the outer structures of her pussy.
- Move up and down the length of the vulva. You can lightly caress the length and width of the vulva from the perineum to the pubic mound. These long and broad strokes will stimulate the entire vulva: outer lips, inner lips, vaginal opening, and clitoris.
- Place your middle finger in the middle vestibule of her pussy, and use your index and ring finger to gently clamp her inner lips against your middle finger. Clamp, pull a bit, and release to give her waves of pleasure. The upper part of your fingers or part of your palm will lie over the clitoris, and you can keep it all locked together and vibrate your hand, moving in all directions. This will work best with a woman who has longer inner lips.
- Clamp the inner lips, clitoris, and shaft between your first two fingers and move them back and forth like you would kick your legs when swimming. You will be stimulating the sides of the clit and shaft, and the inner lips will rub together. This is a good stroke for someone who likes indirect stimulation of the clit, as it focuses on the root and legs of the clitoris.
- Close your fingers and cup them. Use your fingertips turned sideways to touch the inner lips, clitoris, and shaft in a side-to-side movement, like waving sideways over her vulva. Your fingertips will be stimulating the clit and the length of the inner lips with this gentle motion.
- Spread her inner lips open with your index and ring finger while running your middle finger up and down the inner vestibule in long strokes from the bottom all the way up to the clit.
- Stimulate her vaginal entrance. Don't just go in without giving it a second thought—remember to tease. Stimulate

the outside, circle around it, and explore the form of the opening. If you penetrate her, build up to it, make her want it, and choose the perfect moment to go in.

- If you are really dexterous and your hand size matches her vulva well, you can penetrate her vagina with, say, your middle finger while your thumb maintains a consistent rhythm on her clit. This one really takes some coordination, but if she likes penetration and you get it just right, she will be most grateful for your effort.

- Spend some time caressing the anus with a finger, making small circles around its opening (with some lube), and continue the circular motion or do some mini-thrusts into it. Remember not to use that finger on her vulva again until it is thoroughly washed (more on that in "Ass-istance for Two" in "The Ins and Outs" chapter).

- Stimulate her perineum (the spot between the vulva and the anus) with firm up-and-down or circular motions.

- Pinch the inner lips and tug on them. If she likes it a little bit rougher and likes the stinging sensation of pinching, she might dig this one.

Play with the pressure and rhythm of these strokes. Use them in any combination, or create your own. Follow her lead, and she might show you one you wouldn't have thought of. You can teasingly graze the vulvic surface or apply more pressure. You can slow down and tease, finger, or caress any area that gives her pleasure.

Talk the Talk, Walk the Walk

Patience and practice are the keys to becoming a digital master. A clit, although in some ways similar, is not a dick, so don't treat it like one. And don't forget the basics. Have your lover take your fingers on a walk and ask her what she likes, then give it a try. Getting to know where and how your lover likes to be touched takes time. In the process, you might discover some new things. One day she'll give you one of the biggest compliments a lover can give: "He really knows my body. He knows exactly how to touch me."

There is a great way to find out how your lover likes to be touched: Ask her. Hearken back to the show 'n' tell piece in the last chapter. If you don't know how to touch her, or if what you are doing doesn't seem to be working, ask her to show you— and take copious mental notes. You can even place your hand lightly over hers to follow the motion she makes.

When you're learning to digitally co-pilot, it's important to keep a few things in mind. Does she have a favorite side of her clitoris? A lot of women do. Does she like to be stimulated lower or higher on her shaft? Does she home in on one area and stay with it, or does she move around the entire vulva? How does she stimulate her clit? Does she touch it directly or indirectly, back and forth, side to side, in a circular or diagonal motion? Does she tap or stroke? Grind or graze? This information is crucial and can really help you out, so pay attention!

☀ The Lowdown on Going Down

When it comes to cunnilingus, most men suck! Many heterosexual women we surveyed testified that really great head is hard to come by.

What is it about cunnilingus that is so intimidating? Well, for one thing, it's incredibly intimate. There you are at the gateway to the tunnel of love, where all the smells, secretions, and every tiny little movement is, well, in your face! That's as intense for the one getting it as it is for the one giving it. When it comes to going down, almost everyone could use a little heads-up advice.

Loving It

I love to go down on a woman because it tastes good, it feels good on my lips and tongue, and I love having my head between a woman's legs and feeling her writhe while listening to her moan. —Katie, 28, Portland, Oregon

Before I had been with women sexually, all I could fanta-size about was how amazing it would be to suck on a woman's pussy. And when I finally got to do it, it was hot-ter than I ever could have imagined.

—Terry, 29, San Francisco

With guys, there seem to be two camps when it comes to cunnilingus: those who like to go down and those who don't. The same goes for lesbians. But since cunnilingus is such an im-portant part of lesbian sex, more gay women are comfortable with it and consequently more skilled.

Just as you guys love a woman who enjoys going down on you, women love men who enjoy going down on them.

I once asked the woman in my life who gave far and away the best head I'd ever experienced how she got so good. Her answer was very simple: "I just love to do it."

—Jim, 28, Boston

You're usually going to be pretty good at doing what you love—at least you'll bring desire and passion to it. So if you're in the camp that doesn't have a sweet love affair with cunnilingus, re-member that many great things in life are acquired tastes: caviar, fine scotch, wine, classical music, and cunnilingus.

What the Men Say

- I love a woman who likes to give a blow job. I love this not simply because it feels good, but because it's in-credibly intimate.
- It's all trust, man. My most vulnerable and sensitive appendage is being surrounded by her teeth and jaws. Giving a blow job makes a woman powerful.
- Beyond the physical pleasure, she is also validat-ing . . . no, much more than that, worshipping my cock, giving it her full attention. She's loving it.

It's clear that for most men a blow job is more than just a blow job. It's about intimacy, trust, and, if you're fortunate enough, a dollop of worship. We all need these things, especially from our lovers.

When you go down on a woman, it's about a whole lot more than an orgasm. It makes a woman feel good all over—clit, body, mind, and spirit. If you don't give her that attention, she will feel something is missing. She will feel her sacred space has not been given the love and attention it deserves. She likes a little worship, too. This type of attention is especially important for women, because most don't reach orgasm through intercourse as easily as you guys, who can usually count on some good old-fashioned deep thrusting to get you off.

So get ready to dive in!

In the Mood

Male or female, no one is *always* in the mood to eat pussy or suck dick. If you're not, be honest with yourself and your partner and ask for a raincheck. But if you're *never* in the mood, then you have other issues to work on, because this is one of the tastiest layers of sex cake for women. It's hard to be horny and motivated on cue, especially after a hard day at work, but it's important to make the effort. Think how you would feel if she was never in the mood for your favorite sexual act.

On the other hand, she may not always want oral sex either. If you are a cunnilingus aficionado, it could be disappointing if she doesn't want your mouth on her pussy. Oral sex is complicated. It takes a lot of trust—allowing someone to taste one's most personal or private bodily region—and surrender to allow someone to perform this intimate act. Many people find oral sex to be more intimate than intercourse. If she's not in the mood for it, don't push. She's not going to be open to what you are working so hard to provide. If she's *never* in the mood and never allows you to go down on her, she probably has bigger issues that need to be dealt with. Maybe she is uncomfortable with the way her vulva looks or smells and is afraid to share it with you so closely. Or maybe she's had bad experiences with oral sex in the past.

It would be helpful to be sensitive to her feelings and initiate a dialogue about it. Ask her questions in a gentle manner that will help her open up about her issues. If you haven't built enough trust with her, she probably won't engage, but if you have, you could help her learn to love her genitals or work through whatever issues are coming up for her. Then, hopefully, you'll both be in the mood.

The Par-clit-ulars

Getting to know her clit, getting to know all about it . . .

Sex isn't like driving an old Buick. We're all built for performance when it comes to sex. And we each come with our own personalized owner's manual. There are no short cuts in the journey of discovering what drives your lover wild, but first you have to know the basics. Hopefully, you weren't a bad boy and you read the anatomy chapter. If you didn't, stop right now, go back, and read it, or else you'll be punished, and so will your next lover. Learn it, know it, love it!

> *I knew a "bi" girl who generously offered herself up to a sweet but nerdy late-blooming college boy. When he realized that he could have at it down there with an uninhibited woman who really loved her body, he actually jumped out of bed, ran to a desk drawer, and grabbed a magnifying glass, the better to finally study the exotic land of VULVA, the eighth wonder of the world.* —Anonymous

Since a woman's center of pleasure is her clitoris, oral sex is one of the most surefire ways for her to reach orgasm. Clits are very particular. They are finely tuned instruments of pleasure that need to be played in the right way. And if you can't give it to 'em that way, then move over, 'cause the vibrator is just on the other side of the bed. Read on and you won't suffer that fate.

> :♡: **Honey, Come Closer**
>
> Get your whole mouth around her clit and suck on it like the luscious fruit it is. Don't be shy. Don't just flick it with your tongue. How would you like it if she never made full contact with your dick?

Every woman likes something different, but there are a few tricks you should know, and a little practice makes puurrrfect.

Overcoming Porno Tongue

> *My most important sexual teacher was porno movies, because you can see all the tricks of the trade displayed for you like an educational video.* —Bob, 21, Brooklyn

If you've been learning how to go down from pornos, here's a key thing to remember: Those shots of women going down on women or men going down on women are all staged for the camera, for the viewer jacking off at home—not for the pleasure of the woman who is receiving the cunnilingus. You see those sideways poses with the tongue sticking out inches away from target, and since porn viewers have short attention spans, the woman usually gets about thirty seconds of tongue before the stud moves to some other body part. Or she has one of those screaming fake porno orgasms.

So men learn to perform a kind of stiff-tongued, long-distance, mechanical flickfest while the woman lies there bored and frustrated, counting tongue strokes instead of sheep!

Do not mimic porno tongue. Your tongue should not be stretched as far out as possible, giving the absolute minimum of contact with her pussy. Grazing over the surface of her clit in short, pithy, frustrating strokes will not get you a gold star. You need to get your whole mouth and her whole vulva involved.

Rule of Tongue

In dealing with the clitoris, the buildup is crucial. Okay, the clitoris *is* the bull's-eye. But it's vitally important to stimulate all the wider circles that lead to the center. Learn to slow down. What's the rush? The more you immerse yourself, the more you will both experience! Eating pussy is like a memorable road trip. It's not the destination that counts, it's the journey.

> ### ☼♡☼ Honey, Come Closer
>
> Work your way slowly to the clit. Start with the outer regions first—the inner thighs, inner and outer lips. Go the length and width of the vulva. You get the picture. Don't just zip to the clit like it's a bull's-eye.

Tease her first. Breathe hard on her vulva, kiss it all over, everywhere but her clitoris. Kiss her thighs and belly, continue to tease, tease, tease, work up, finally kiss her clit, move away, and come back. Play with her. Have fun with it. Start licking with nice long strokes, feeling out the whole vulva—the lips, the shaft, the vaginal entryway. Work your way to the bull's-eye. Once you're in there, explore. Spend some time on the shaft, then run your tongue down each side of her clit and tickle it underneath. Start with light, teasing caresses. Don't miss any of the terrain. Swirl your tongue around the hood, circumscribing the love button. Then get your whole mouth around her clitoris. Kiss it with deep French swirl clit kisses. Suck it if she can handle that much stimulation. Give the clit the great blow job you've always dreamed of.

The clitoris is very sensitive. Any extra stimulation (fingers, faster rhythm, or more pressure) could ruin her buildup. A clitoris doesn't respond like a penis. It doesn't necessarily want harder and faster as orgasm approaches. If it ain't broke, don't fix it. Don't go faster. Don't lick harder. Just get in touch with your inner drummer and keep the steady beat, man.

:♡: **Honey, Come Closer**

If her clit is hard and she's getting into a groove, don't destroy the rhythm of the clitoral stimulation! If it's work- ing for her, *keep doing it.* If your partner is getting really hot, moaning, breathing hard, getting sweaty, moving her hips into you, or saying something like "Oh yes! Oh god yes! Yes, right there! Ohmigod! Yeeeessss!" then just keep doing whatever it is you're doing. This is *not* a signal to increase speed or pressure.

Communicating Orally

Pay attention to the way she moves. Is she rocking her hips back and forth? Is she pushing harder into your mouth? Is she pulling away? Is she wincing? If you're unsure, ask. Come up for air and ask specific questions: "Is this the right pressure? Do you want me to go faster? Harder? Softer?" Then do it. Better to know what she wants than to keep doing something that isn't work- ing. Be specific. If you simply say, "Is this okay?" or some other general inquiry, she may not feel like she can tell you the truth, or it may require too much of a break in the action to explain. You could have her show you that special area she wants you to focus on. If you are one of those guys who hates being ex- pected to be a mind reader, then you know the value of com- munication about such delicate matters!

Be a Good Sport

I wish men understood that not only is the clitoris impor- tant in stimulating a woman to reach an orgasm, but that it may take a while to get there and not to give up after a few minutes, thinking that was enough to satisfy her.
—Tonya, 26, Bryan, Texas

For a great cunnilingus session, you've got to be prepared to go the distance. Be ready for fifteen rounds if necessary. Don't think you're going to be down there for a few minutes and she'll explode in a mind-blowing orgasm, then beg you to bang her afterward. You have a better chance of being the next ambassador to the isle of Lesbos. Effortless, easy, mind-blowing orgasms can happen, but for most women they take time and conscious effort. So be patient and giving. She'll love you for it. A good work ethic is an important part of giving great head. All great athletes are willing to stay after practice and do that extra lap!

Coming Up for Air

So you've been down there awhile and your tongue needs a little breather. You can do this without taking a commercial break at the climactic moment in the drama. One thing you can do is use your fingers on her clit for a couple of minutes while your tongue rests and recharges. You have to do this with some finesse, though. Try to match the pressure and rhythm of your tongue with your fingers. This can be difficult to gauge, since our tongues and fingers have different levels of sensitivity. Lick your fingers first or swirl up some pussy juice. If you're really good, she won't know the difference. But if she's edging on orgasm, huffing and puffing, ready to fly through the roof, stay with your tongue, reach deep inside yourself, and find a second or third wind to blow the roof off.

Be a Poet

Then there's the question of style. Who teaches a man to go down on a woman? Unless a guy is lucky enough to hang out with lesbians or have a really terrific relationship with a woman who's open to mutual exploration, communication, and experimentation, he finds himself forced to perform without ever having a great coach.

What's it supposed to be like? If you really want to charm and satisfy the ladies, you need to become a poet: sensuous, open, creator of rhythm and sound.

Imagine a sweet, satiny cave of nooks and crannies,
Where every fold and texture
Is sensitive to every touch and tug
And stroke and nibble of
Your handsome mug.
Now imagine where all the lips meet,
A fat, ripe strawberry
Soaked in Grand Marnier, as you tongue
And suck every drop of sweet liqueur
Without bruising the berry,
Swirling and slurping her swollen sweet, wild,
Deep rooted, blood-ripe, fleshy fruit
That's always in season.

Get the idea? So dive in and let the poet in you come out. We're talking an inspired jazz riff, a deep bass chord, an amazing rhyme, a lush glass of wine you want to savor to the last sip, or a poem to melt her with. Set your pussy poet free.

Talking Taste and Smell

Lesbian women are less shy when it comes to talking about taste, smell, and their cycle. Unfortunately, we live in a culture that promotes self-improvement products for everything, especially things that don't need improvement. Pussies fall within this you're-not-okay-just-the-way-you-are category. Don't buy into our culture's dysfunctions. "Mom, some days I just don't feel fresh. What do I do?" Remember that one? There are a thousand and one fresh scents for pussies. Well, guess what? Chemicals, douches, and feminine-hygiene sprays don't go well with pussy. They mess with the vulva's natural flavor and scent, balance and health. Douching is actually bad for vaginas, and can cause problems by upsetting the natural pH balance. Vaginas have mechanisms to clean themselves, and douches get in the way of that. They're not good for you either. Try licking your underarm after you've sprayed it with Right Guard.

So please don't add to this ridiculous pressure on women to improve everything about themselves, right down to their genitals, by encouraging your partners to douche. That kind of behavior just plays on women's insecurities. This is not to say that there won't be partners whose taste and smell aren't your favorite weekly special. Or that a partner whose taste and smell you normally love won't have off days. If there is ever a marked change in a woman's genital smell and it's truly unpleasant, that could indicate she has some kind of vaginal infection, and she might want to get it checked out. If you notice this in a partner with whom you have established trust, gently bring it to her attention. Don't forget to make it your practice to tell her you love her taste and smell.

❤ Honey, Come Closer

There is nothing hotter than a partner who loves the way her genitals and juices taste and smell. Not many things will put a woman more at ease for some good lickin' than a partner complimenting how she tastes. Lesbians are pretty good at validating their partners' genital appearance, flavor, and scent. Wouldn't you like a woman to tell you what a nice dick you have and how good it tastes in her mouth? Same idea.

Etiquette for the Orally Challenged

Etiquette is crucial for cunnilingus. This is a touchy subject. Our culture doesn't go out of its way to make women comfortable with their taste and smell. So you need to be her champion. One woman shared the tale of a friend who was having sex with a male partner: He went down on her for a few minutes, then poked his head up and asked if she had a breath mint so he could get the taste out of his mouth! This guy's tongue would be on a chopping block if we could get a hold of it, so he would never be able to wound someone like that again. She may never let another partner go down on her, and she probably spent a fortune on therapy trying to get over that one.

Other no-nos include getting up to brush your teeth as soon as you finish a cunnilingus session. Even if you feel the need, give it a little time. Let the loving linger first, then get up to use the bathroom. If you just can't help yourself and need or want to brush, if you're obsessive-compulsive and constantly wash your hands, or if you suffer from phobias, communicate this to your partner so she knows it's not her. Our lovers appreciate it when we take care of ourselves, just use common sense and be sensitive in your approach.

Positioning

Pillow Prop. Pillows are always a great help. When placed under the woman's bottom, they prop up the pelvis so that you can be comfortable and have easier access. This position is also comfy for your partner. She might want her head propped up as well, for easier communication and the pleasure of watching you eat her.

Have a Seat. It may be more comfortable for you to lie on your back and have your partner straddle you—you know, sit on your face, so to speak. As she faces you, she can lean up against a wall for support, taking some of the stress off her thighs.

On the Edge. Bring your lover to the edge of the bed, with you on your knees on the floor and the object of your desire right in your face. Then push her legs toward her shoulders for easy access.

Changing positions can be helpful for her and for you. It can help you to avoid cricks in your neck and keep body parts from falling asleep. You can always return to your personal favorite.

The State-of-the-Tongue Address

You can make your tongue soft and sloppy or tense and hard. A hard tongue might feel good when you're tongue fucking or stimulating your lover's outer lips, but it might be too abrasive on her clitoris. A hard tongue might feel great on the shaft of her clitoris but too rough on the glans, especially if you've pulled back her hood, exposing her head. She may want you to use your best soft, sloppy tongue for caressing her clit, or if she has a tough li'l clitty, a firm tongue might be just fine. The important thing to remember is that your tongue is capable of variety. So be sure to explore all your options.

Lesbians know that if you want to be a good lover of women, your tongue is one of your greatest physical assets. This is something that penis-centered men don't get. Work it out, strengthen it, and train it to perform well. And for goddess sake, get your whole mouth involved, not just the small area at the tip of your tongue.

For good head, your tongue needs to be patient and strong. The best way to practice your strokes and get in shape is to get a little work in every day with your lover. Practice being delicate yet precise. Try different strokes. Test out the techniques we outline in the pages to follow.

> *When I go down on a woman, it's not just about the clit. I focus on the whole area, building up, working from the thighs in. Suck on the outer lips, then the inner lips, stick my tongue in, maybe brush by the clit and breathe on it. Go back and forth. Variety is good because if you keep doing the same thing all the time, the body gets numb to it or bored. There are points you want to focus on because they're more sensitive, but it's a different kind of sensation when you include everything.*
>
> —Linda, 31, Newport, Rhode Island

Tongue Fucking

A good tongue fucking can be total nirvana. If you've ever been on the receiving end, you know. A soft tongue thrusting in and out of an orifice is a yummy pleasure. It's about being penetrated, probed, and teased with that most facile of organs, the one that feels most at home in a pussy precisely because of its

> ### ✨💓✨ Honey, Come Closer
>
> Tongue fucking is one of the great lost arts. Have fun with it. Lick around the opening, then dart your tongue in, thrusting it as deep as you can. Go slow, go fast, tease her with the tip. Then toss her knees behind her head and give her a tongue fucking she'll never forget. Whatever length, if your tongue is strong and you know how to use it, she will be forever grateful.

moistness and texture. If you don't want to delve quite so deep, give her a nice licking.

The Combo Platter, Please

If she likes penetration, there is nothing like some G-spot stimulation while sucking her clit. After you've warmed her pussy up, you can insert a finger and add another later if she wants, depending on how skilled you are and the positioning of her vulva. Sometimes your hand can get in the way of your mouth and you may need to turn to a 69 position or work on some other fancy maneuvers in order to get to everything. A combo is a little bit like juggling. You have to keep a good rhythm going on her clit while you are fingering her. You can also use a small dildo that would still allow enough room for your mouth if that would please her. Use whatever she likes to be penetrated with. Or try this little trick: Put the vibrator under your tongue as you caress her. This could lead to a screaming ovation if your tongue can handle it.

Anal Play

Another version of the combo platter involves anal stimulation. As always, start slow. While you're going down, start to massage around her sphincter muscle, then give her perineum some nice firm strokes. Now you can slowly insert a lubed finger, just barely entering her at first. Let her sphincter pucker around your finger. That may be enough help to send your lover into orgasm, or she may like your finger to go all the way in. She might like the in-and-out motion nice and easy, or she might like it hard and fast. Maybe she wants more than one finger. Communicate with her. Let her order the combo platter she wants, then serve it up.

Combo Platter Deluxe

You knew it was coming. That's right, stick one finger in her vagina and one finger in her butt. Again, go slowly and don't let your clitoral caresses fall by the wayside. Be careful. There are bacteria in her anus, and her vagina doesn't like them at all! Do not mix up your fingers or allow them to touch, as that could cause a bacterial infection.

Again, make sure you listen to her signals. If she's trying to reach through and pull your hand or dildo out, it may be too much stimulation for her or it may not be what she wants at that moment. If her pleasure sounds decrease or something seems to shift away from pleasure, come up and say, "Do you want me to come out or stay in?" Then she can let you know what she wants at that moment.

Hummers

You may have heard of hummers for men. If you're lucky, you've experienced one. This technique can also drive a woman crazy. It's pretty simple. While sucking and licking, you hum on her vulva and clit, sending sound vibrations via your mouth to her hot spots like a human vibrator. It shows your appreciation. Just the sound of you really getting into it and relishing her genitals can be a huge turn-on. Try it.

Nibble and Flick

To drive your partner wild, use your front teeth to gently get a hold of her clitoris where her shaft meets the head. Keep it anchored with your teeth so it can't wiggle away, and gently flick the head of her clit against the inside of your teeth with your tongue. It's a technique that takes practice, because your tongue can get worn out fast. It is also easier to perform on a woman whose clitoris protrudes a bit.

69

This position has its pros and cons. It's hard to focus fully on your arousal and give your lover your full attention when you're in it, yet it does get both people excited and engaged in an activity that may not be goal-oriented and focusing primarily on the orgasm. As you give each other head simultaneously in a 69 position, the focus shifts to mutually experienced sensations and fun visual angles. It may not be the best position for bringing your lover to orgasm. Many women have to concentrate on their arousal to reach orgasm, working their breathing and their PC muscle. It's pretty hard to do this while wrapping your mouth around another set of genitals. So 69 is a good way to get your motor going, and it's fun to taste and be tasted. And if either of you comes, bonus!

Safer Licking? Dam Her!

Oral sex is usually the behavior that will put lesbians most at risk for STIs. On the hierarchy of bodily-fluid exchange, cunnilingus is not as risky for the giver or receiver as fellatio or vaginal or anal intercourse, but there is still a risk of spreading sexually transmitted infections.

For safer cunnilingus, the best thing we've got to date is dental dams, sometimes called lollies or a host of other names. Basically a dental dam is a thin, flat sheet of latex that you use as a barrier for oral-anal or oral-vulvic contact. What you do is this: Start by putting some lube on her vulva. Don't skimp. Latex on dry clit is about as enjoyable as three months of overdue bills. Then lay the dam over her vulva, hold it in place, and lick away. If you want, you can even add some flavored lube or honey on your side for fun. She can still feel heat through the latex, as well as your strokes. Dental dams are not the most exciting item in the sex world, but they provide protection, and if you can entertain a latex fetish, they are an erotic bonus. Also, for men with harsh stubble or facial hair, a latex barrier may provide a lot more comfort for her sensitive vulva!

Make Your Own Latex Barrier

For a little twist, you can take a latex glove (you know, the ones the doc uses) and make it into a latex barrier. Get as large a glove as you can get and get some scissors that cut well, then:

1. Cut the four fingers off the glove at their base. Make sure you leave the thumb!
2. Cut lengthwise all the way up the side of the glove where the outside of your hand would be.
3. Open it up and voilà! You have a latex barrier for cunnilingus or analingus with a special thumb-shaped attachment you can put inside the orifice of choice for deeper licking! You can also cut a condom lengthwise and open it up for a small latex barrier. Just make sure it isn't lubricated with spermicide. You don't want a numb mouth!

A Quick Oral Review

- Start easy, tease, go slow, and work up speed and pressure according to what your partner likes.
- Communicate with *specific* inquiries. Remember, with clitorises, you have to be on target. This isn't horseshoes.
- Make sure to keep the lines of communication open so she can tell you what she wants. Encourage her to let you know how she feels and what she likes.
- If you have facial hair, go with the grain. Stubble and vulvas do not mix. Chafed vulvas are no fun. A latex barrier will help.

- Use your whole mouth, not just the tip of your tongue. Forget the big-money tongue shots in porn.
- Strengthen your tongue. Exercise that muscle! Practice makes perfect.
- If she's getting really excited, *don't* change what you're doing. Just keep doing it!
- Don't stop until she wants you to.

The Ins
and Outs

☀ Another Course in Intercourse

Vaginal sex is not the staple of my sexual relationships. It's one of many things. I first ask my lover what kind of vaginal penetration she likes, and then we go from there. She might want different things, and there are many ways to meet her needs. Mix it up, that's the key. I like to try different things and see how they feel. —Lydia, 27, Philadelphia

Lesbians approach vaginal intercourse differently from most men. For them, it is but one element of the experience rather than the pinnacle of it. This orientation allows them to take their time and enjoy the ride more, not necessarily pushing to orgasm because that can happen in myriad ways. If you already experience vaginal intercourse in this way, kudos to you. If not, try to shift the way you see and do it. Many women complain that sex usually ends when their male partner comes, and they are left unsatisfied. Don't be one of those guys who roll over and go to sleep in typical self-serving fashion. Make sure your lover gets all she wants and needs too. You should both have an experience that feels great.

You may be wondering what lesbians can possibly teach you about vaginal intercourse. Plenty, honey. There are many lesbians who enjoy using a dildo or other toys for vaginal penetration. Be assured, many lesbians have had intercourse with men as well as women.

Intercourse Basics

For most women, intercourse is not the primary way to have orgasms. Many women love to fuck, but only about thirty percent have orgasms that way. Take two things from this. One, intercourse cannot be the alpha and omega of your sexual repertoire. Two, don't feel like a loser if your lover doesn't have an orgasm every time you have intercourse. Don't base success and failure on orgasm count. Base it on how you feel as a whole person. Did you have an emotional and physical release? Do you feel connected and open toward your partner? Do you feel like you've just been on a fun journey? Were you a good lover? Did you bring good energy? Were you generous and giving? Were you fully present? If you and your partner have answered yes to these questions, you're living the good life, soaking up the many positive benefits of sex.

It's also crucial that you and your partner are using condoms for any type of intercourse. If you choose not to, then you should decide together before you get naked so both of you are clear about what risks you are taking and how you will proceed. If you or your partner is worried about getting an STI for any part of your sexual encounter, the whole thing will suffer and that's no fun for anyone. Worry does not make for good sex, and not using a condom does not make you an attentive or responsive lover. So nip that one in the bud, so to speak, and keep the latex handy. Even lesbians use them on their dildos!

Intercourse is a lot like a dance. You need to know some basic steps. You need the skills to take the lead and the confidence to surrender. Then you can groove on all levels.

Getting Inside: The Gift of Pussy

It's hard to describe, but it's all about trust, connection, and surrender. Oh yeah, let's not forget surrender.
—Terri, 30, Pittsburgh

*I always feel like I'm sharing something really sacred with
a partner. There is nothing more vulnerable than someone
physically entering your body with theirs. I love the way it
fills me up. If I have a real emotional connection to a partner, which I've realized is more and more important the
older I get, then the intensity of him or her entering me can
be overwhelming sometimes—in a good way.*
—Anisa, 27, Lakewood, California

*If it involves my body part going inside someone, I treat that
as really special. It's really intense to have that kind of
power with penetration, whether it's fingers, dildos, fists. It's
a really vulnerable thing to open up your body to someone.*
—Anne, 29, Dallas

When you enter your lover's pussy, you pass beyond the
threshold of the mundane world into her sacred temple. That is
an honor and a privilege. A gift. Lesbians often have a greater
consciousness of what it means to enter a woman's pussy because
they have one too. If you have taken this for granted before, rethink that attitude. Would you take lightly allowing someone to
penetrate you, to enter your anus, to fuck you, to be inside your
body? Probably not. Most heterosexual men take that kind of
thing very seriously. Approach any penetration of her pussy
with reverence, be it with fingers, toys, objects, or your cock.
When honored and respected, this warm, lush place will embrace you with love and desire.

*The first time I was with my first girlfriend, she asked me if
she could go inside me. I was floored, hardly knowing how
to respond. No man had ever asked permission before . . .
they had all just assumed they could go in there. That was
a turning point for me, to have the power to give permission
for entry. It was so fucking hot when she asked and waited
for my reply instead of just forcing her way in. "Yes," I*

said. "Oh, yes, please come inside," I invited her, my heart pounding with my excitement. My anticipation was heightened, and so was the experience of her being inside me.
                                                    —Dana, 25, Brooklyn

Ask her if you can enter her. Don't assume you have free rein just because she's aroused, or you are, or because you've been in there before. If she doesn't want you in there, it is her right to keep you out. Respect it. She might not want to be entered that day, and some women do not like penetration at all. Far too many women have been penetrated unwillingly at some point in their lives. That kind of abuse will always be in their psyches. For someone to come along and give the power back to her— if she has not already taken it back herself—is a redeeming act. If she thinks it's weird that you are asking, that's probably because *nobody* has ever bothered to ask, and she's probably never empowered herself to be able to decide whether she wants a lover inside her or not. You will get ten gold stars for that display of respect for her desires and boundaries.

ː♡ː Honey, Come Closer

Many women who have sex with women know how precious the act of entering a woman's vagina is and will ask, "Can I go inside you?" That's one of the sexiest things you can say, placing the power to say yes or no back where it belongs—with the person who owns the orifice.

The power she feels when she's asked permission will directly correlate to her enjoyment of the experience. We need lots of sexual healing, and it begins with both men and women respecting the sacredness in each of our bodies and the value of choosing to share them. If you ask and she says no for any reason, then do other things to make you both happy.

Penetration vs. Thrusting

First, let's get our definitions straight: Penetration and thrust-ing are not the same thing. Penetration is about trust, surrender, a give-and-take, and shifting roles regardless of gender combi-nation. There is no way to avoid the energy that will infuse the act of penetration. A woman is receiving, allowing, taking in, while her partner is entering, inserting, servicing. It can be rough, or it can be gentle. Either way, it is about the physical, psychological, and energetic entrance into a private, special place. It is, after all, the inside of her body. That's about as pri-vate and intimate as you can get.

Thrusting, on the other hand, is about sensation. It's about wanting to go wild with pleasure. Thrusting is about giving pleas-ure, and if it's done well, you might get an invitation to come back. When you're inside your lover, pay attention to her nipple texture, the changes in body flush, the movement of breath, how her hips move. Is she grabbing and squeezing you? Is she un-controllably spanking you? If you're lucky. Or talented. Don't lose track of these details because you are thinking about your own dick, performance, and pleasure.

What feels best to men is often hard, rhythmic thrusting, es-pecially as they near orgasm. This may or may not be what she likes. You need to find her rhythm, not yours, since her pussy will probably be more particular than your dick for pleasure and comfort's sake.

Because of the mixed bag of emotional, cultural, physical, and psychological factors that converge during intercourse, there needs to be a symphonic flow to the art of thrusting. A man may just want to go deep, deeper, deepest until he comes. For a woman, the experience of sensation from a variety of rhythms and movements may be erotic, and far more exciting to her than fifteen minutes of pneumatic drilling.

Moving In

You've asked your partner if you can enter her and she let out a gaspy "yes, please." The first step is to get in with grace and love. This is not as easy as it sounds, and the first dip into the pool of love is one of the most powerful and crucial moments of intercourse.

When it comes to penetrating, there are no hard-and-fast rules about who should do it. A lot depends on the nature of the relationship.

> *Once I was dating this butch, and the first time she fucked me with her cock, I reached down to put it inside because I'm so used to helping out male partners. She stopped me, pulled my hand off her cock, and said, "I'll do that," with a firm confidence that got me so wet I couldn't wait another second for her to enter me and fuck me real good.*
> —Jeanine, 35, West Hollywood, California

Many women prefer to guide the penetration, especially if they need you to ease in, because they can control how much and how fast. The woman-on-top position is good for this. When she is the one inserting, learn from her. How does she do it? Does she use two hands? Maybe she controls your cock with one hand, spreads her inner lips with the other if need be, then eases it in. This is your first lesson: Use two hands. She's also probably pretty smooth about it and does it in one fell swoop. That's your second lesson: Don't panic, and take your time.

When you are on top, it can be difficult to find the much-sought-after entrance, because you can't see it. When you bend your neck to look down, you see her stomach and her pubic hair. It's a beautiful sight but not very helpful for the task at hand. It is also difficult to use two hands if you need them to prop yourself up. From the missionary position, a good way to penetrate your lover is to sit up between her legs so you can see what you are doing. Sit back on your haunches and scoot your hips in close to her, sliding your knees and thighs under her spread legs. It's not as complicated as it sounds. Open her lips with one hand and slide your cock in with the other.

spread legs. It's not as complicated as it sounds. Open her lips with one hand and slide your cock in with the other.

Moment of Entry—Make It Last

> *I like him to put it in so he can tease me and I don't know
> when it's going to happen.*   —Tracy, 33, New York

Women know how to be teases; you can be too. Don't rush to the game's end by going for the hole-in-one with one swipe of your club. Build up, child, build up. Use the head of your penis to massage her clit. Take your dick and rub it in between her inner lips, running the head up and down the length of her pussy without penetrating. Feel her wet juices on your glans. If you don't feel some juice, she might not be ready. If she is mentally ready to fuck but isn't physically wet, grab the lube. Put some on your cock, stroke it all over the shaft and head, then spread the rest on her pussy with a nice caress of your hand.

Keep teasing her with your cock. Make her want it so bad she's practically pushing her pussy up around your member. Pause at her vaginal opening, circle around it a bit, pause some more, then stick it in just a millimeter, like you're finally going to enter her, then pull it away.

You can also seductively stroke yourself so that you stay hard. A lot of men rush to penetrate because they fear they'll lose their hard-on. Now you're in control. No worries. Take your time and enjoy the view.

☼♡☼ Honey, Come Closer

By taking your time, not only do you create steamy anticipation in your partner; you also get to check out the territory and get a good sense of where everything is so there is no clumsy fumbling when you do finally enter her. Learn to slow down.

*I like her to tease me and enter real slow so I can savor
every inch.*   —Kelly, 31, Minneapolis

When you've teased her (and yourself) enough, enter her as
slowly and tenderly or as rough and furiously as the moment
dictates. At first, it's best to go slow, unless she forces your dick
in her because she wants it so bad—all lubed up and ready to
take the entire thing. As you start to penetrate, be sensitive to
how easily you slide in. Make a moment of it. Pause, take a
breath, and look her in the eye. Dante knew the power of the
gaze when he spoke of Beatrice and said, "She shot arrows out
of her eyes into my heart." Look for signs of pleasure, moaning,
her hips rising to take more of you or rocking toward you.
Sometimes sounds of pain and pleasure are similar. If you are
confused, check in and ask her if this is okay. Don't force it. If
it's still not silky smooth, pull out and get her juiced up. A little
oral stimulation is usually effective.

☙ Honey, Come Closer

It's always a good idea to lick her pussy and get it all
hot and horny before trying to put your penis in it. She'll
be juicy and swollen, and intercourse will be a lot more
comfortable.

Role Models

Thrusting is a skill. Chances are, what feels best to you will
not be the most enjoyable thing for her, and maybe you've never
had a reputable role model show you how. Find out what she
likes. Asking her in a serious, sultry tone *how* she would like to
be fucked might be the second-hottest question you could ask
her. Now, that's foreplay! She might be dumbfounded that you
asked. She might not know how she wants to be fucked. Or she
may know *exactly* how, and you will have given her the perfect
opportunity to tell you so that you can deliver the goods. As you
go, ask her what positions or angles feel good to her. Ask her

which parts of her vagina are most sensitive. These are things you need to know, and most of us didn't have very good thrusting role models to show and tell us. It was either porn dude or one of our best friends.

> *My first lesson in fucking happened in my friend Chuck's backyard. Me and Chuck were in sixth grade and we watched his two dogs do it. We were both wide-eyed, watching Sparky hump Misty. I thought, "My God, one day I'll be doing this." Not with a dog, of course. For years, my sexual mentor was Sparky. I would thrust away at my girlfriends like a wild dog who was six months overdue for his distemper shot.* —Kevin, 32, Houston

In American culture, role-model progression may easily go from the neighbor's dog to porn. What's wrong with this picture? For starters, the big dog on top doesn't care about the other dog's pleasure. In pornos, at least, you actually get to watch real humans fuck, but still, it usually isn't that different from the dogs. They do change rhythms and positions (often like acrobats), and maybe they show a little concern for their partner's pleasure, but rarely do the women have real orgasms, and they always leave out crucial details, like lube!

Some men think of "manly sex" as lots of deep, powerful thrusting. This is how "real men" fuck, right? There is a place for this, and a lot of women really like it, but that's not all they like, and that's not all they want. This is Sparky's technique. Sure, we are animals, and sometimes we will dig into our animal instinct. But if Sparky engaged in a little shallow pussy play, all the female dogs would be jumping his fence.

Know Thyself

Regardless of sexual orientation, two things make a great lover: self-knowledge and knowing what turns your lover on. Now let's focus on you and your technique. You know what works best for your dick. For some men, being in one position or another will help them control the duration of their erection better. Some positions allow for easier muscle control. Some are good for deeper penetration, some better for shallow fucking, while some stimulate her G-spot better. Learn to slow down. Lesbians have some advantages in this area because they can fuck for a while, take a break, come back and mix it up as they wish. No worries about depleted erections. Learn to mix it up. Check in to see what she likes or wants at that moment.

Here are some useful hints to file away so you can call on them for each new partner's varied needs.

The Comfort Factor

Little things can enhance you and your partner's comfort and also make sex hotter. One simple thing is the use of pillows. Prop a couple pillows under your lover's hips when she's on the bottom. If you're doing her doggie style, pillows under her abdomen may help her relax, or you can just bend her over the bed, the desk, or another object of appropriate height. If the bed is high, the height may make it smooth sailing for you, since all you have to do is stand up and focus on the fucking and she can lie comfortably, arms outstretched.

Another thing to be aware of with comfort is that too much hard thrusting against her pelvis can leave it bruised and sore. The best way to minimize this is through check-ins with your lover.

Let's not forget safety. Many lesbians take care to use condoms on their dildos. Safety and condom use should be of utmost importance for you. Part of comfort is safety. If you or your partner is worried about a condom breaking or about the absence or poor use of one, sex won't be very enjoyable or comfortable.

Positions Galore

The not-so-hidden agenda of this chapter is to help you look at intercourse in a new way, not to illustrate ninety-nine different sexual positions. But it *is* important to realize that there are a lot of fun, playful, and potentially exciting positions to explore. One of the best parts of sex is the exploration. It's discovering what turns you on, finding your "hot spots," and finding what turns on your lover. Not everything will. The important thing is checking out the possibilities and having fun doing it, not feeling like every single thing you do must be mind-blowing.

So here's a quick overview. Positions come in six basic categories: man on top, woman on top, side by side, from the rear (The Sparky Special), sitting, and standing. So either buy one of those books that detail all the variations or just play around with them. But don't mistake acrobatics and performance for great sex.

Let Her Ride You

Many women prefer to be on top because it allows them to control the depth, speed, pressure, and clitoral positioning much better. She'll often get more pleasure from being in the driver's seat, and all you have to do is lie back and watch her while you both enjoy the ride.

Together or Apart

When a woman has her legs together while you are thrusting, it makes for a tighter fit. This increases movement of her inner lips, which could mean more clitoral stimulation, depending on her vulva.

⛧♡⛧ Honey, Come Closer

Some women have larger clitorises, or their clits stick out more, which allows for clitoral stimulation from your penis as it thrusts in and out. Some angles will be more optimal for that clitoral contact, so experiment. Not all women will be able to get clitoral stimulation this way, so you will need to use fingers or a vibrator and get the clitoris involved through other means.

Biomechanics of Thrusting

With thrusting, there is the potential for a variety of strokes, deep and shallow, and the opportunity for clitoral stimulation, depending on leg positioning. Is it nobler to go slow, or take up arms and thrust like your life depends upon it? The variations you choose depend on your lover and your moods.

Remember, the most sensitive part of a woman's vagina is the outer two inches. This means you can give a woman a lot of intense pleasure by penetrating her with just the head of your penis. That may be all she wants. The first two inches also become the tightest part of the vagina during intercourse, because they swell with blood. The disciplined skill of slow, shallow fucking is a lost art. Rediscover it.

Shallow. If you are facing each other and your partner's legs are extended straight out, you will not be able to penetrate as deeply, the penetration will be more shallow, while the friction of your pelvis might rub her clit more. If she is on top, she can control how deep or shallow you go, but go easy from underneath and don't push it too much. A side-by-side position— spoon fashion, with you at the back—may also provide the shallow penetration she wants. Her butt cheeks can add some friction for the exposed parts of your penis.

Deep. If you are on top and your partner bends her knees, placing her feet on the bed, floor, or beach towel, you can penetrate her more deeply. With her feet planted, she can also rise up to meet you, which activates her pelvis more rather than keeping it locked stationary. This position is good for some bump-and-grind action, and you are still in a pretty good position for clitoral contact. But you have to work to keep your pubic mounds in touch while you thrust. Just be careful about the pressure you put on her pelvis, or she'll have a sore, bruised pubic bone afterward. A sitting position provides for a cozy embrace and allows you to kiss and get some deeper thrusting in. If you are pretty strong and coordinated, you can also try a standing position, with her against a wall, on a counter or high piece of furniture, or wrapping her legs around your waist. Standing up to fuck always makes for good variety.

Deepest. Deep thrusting is good only if your lover likes contact in the back part of her vagina and pressure on her cervix. Rear entry is one of the best positions for deep thrusting, and you might like the view. However, it doesn't allow you to look at each other, kiss, or have much other bodily contact. With you on top, your partner can take her feet off the bed and bring her knees toward her chest so you can go really deep. In this position, you won't have clitoral stimulation from body friction while you're thrusting, but there will be enough space between you for either of you to stimulate her clit manually. It will be easier for her to do it, since she won't have to hold herself up with her arms. For even deeper penetration, use your arms to bring her knees to her ears and her hips off the ground, or sit up, let her kick up her helium heels, and hold her ankles. When her knees are back, her pelvis tilts, so she gets better G-spot contact as well. If she is on top, she can sit all the way down on your penis and rock away. If she leans back her G-spot may get more stimulation.

Juggling: Adding a Little Finger Love

Can you walk and chew gum at the same time? Stimulating her clit during intercourse is always a good choice. This can be done in a variety of ways from a variety of positions, and it doesn't even have to be done by you. This is one thing lesbians make no bones about.

If you are in a position to provide some steady manual stimulation, do so. If you can't reach her clit, or want to encourage her to stimulate it herself, gently take her hand and put it on her vulva, move it around, then take yours away and let her go solo. You can also engage in a little perineal or anal play. Use all the techniques and sensitivity you learned in the "Finger Love" section of the "Sapphic Arts" chapter to give her pleasureful, consistent manual stimulation. You can also feel free to use toys for stimulation during intercourse.

Applying the Knowledge

How can I stimulate my partner's G-spot during intercourse?

There are several ways to hit this spicy spot during intercourse. Rear entry, or doggie style, allows for deep thrusting while also stimulating the G-spot. While this position can be fun, it is important to check in with your partner about lubrication and arm or knee fatigue. If she wants the combo platter, she can prop a vibrator on a pillow underneath her to stimulate her clit as well. Another position for the G-spot turn-on is to have her sit on your lap and face each other while she leans back a bit and rocks back and forth.

I have a long penis, and my partner finds deep penetration uncomfortable. What is the best position?

You don't have to be hung like a horse to have this problem. Let her be on top so she can control how far into her your penis goes. Or you can lie face-to-face and both extend your legs straight out. A side-to-side position would also be better for shallow fucking. If you are both sitting up, let her control the action. Some women are uncomfortable with any kind of deep penetration, so choose a position that suits her needs.

If my penis isn't long but my partner likes deep penetration, what should I do?

Doggie style would be an optimal position, and the more she arches her back, opening her pussy to you, the farther in you can go. If you want to be able to face each other, either let her be on top, or bring her knees to her ears and thrust away. Sitting up might also work. However you do it, if you are attentive to her clitoris and other areas of pleasure, it should be enjoyable for you both.

Regardless of position, it is important to find angles and creative ways to keep in touch with her clit and to stimulate the internal vaginal areas that arouse her.

Get Playful

Here are a few little penetration games you can play to encourage some mutual giggles or to shift the pace.

Now You See Me, Now You Don't. This is a shallow-sex game you play with the head of your penis. Sitting up and kneeling on your haunches between her legs, you barely go inside her, swirl the head around, then pull out and use the wet head to rub her clit in a swirly motion. Do it again and again. Do your best dick tease!

The Still Pond. Intercourse does not always have to be thrusting. Even good ol' Sparky slows down every now and then. Total stillness is worth exploring. You want to lay bodies together with as much body contact as possible. It's simple yet complex, like a Zen koan, like one hand clapping, like meditating. You are inside her and you both remain completely still, tuning in to each other's body. Listen to her breathing, feel her chest rise and fall, notice her inhale and exhale, notice your own breathing. Pay close attention to how it feels to be inside her. Feel every inch of your penis. Try to feel her heart beat against your body. Let all thoughts and worries go. Be in the moment with all of your senses alive. Let the intensity of feeling build. Your breath might even begin to match each other's. Maybe you'll have an orgasm. Maybe when you start to move it will be like you just returned from Shangri-La. Maybe you'll fall asleep. What could be more peaceful and comforting than falling asleep while inside your lover? This can be a great way to stay connected at the end of a fucking session. Many women will want you to stay inside them, so be still and feel what that's like. As warm and peaceful as this position may be, many women are prone to getting urinary tract infections, and prolonged contact of your penis against her urethra is a risk. Check with your partner about her history of UTIs prior to this exchange. Also, if you are using condoms, this is unsafe, as they will slip off.

Tag Team. This is a game where you switch off between intercourse and another fun activity. Oral sex is a great choice. Go from fucking to going down on her, from fucking to her blowing you, from fucking to toys and back again. From intercourse to a sweet or nasty spanking, "Tag, you're it!"

Body Rub

Many body parts can stimulate your partner, even to orgasm. Connecting with these other body parts can be just as intimate and satisfying as what you normally think of as intercourse. Lesbians use their thighs, their hips, their breasts, and their butts to stimulate their partner's vulva. You can do the same thing. Lesbians spend a lot of time rubbing bodies and genitals and enjoying the pleasure it provides. Many women have orgasms this way. You can use other body parts besides your penis to stimulate her. Have your lover ride your thigh or your butt. Use your chest to stimulate her pussy. Body rubbing can be one of the most sensual elements of any sexual encounter. Spend some time on the outside before you venture in. It's a way to connect and awaken your bodies, so get your whole body involved.

Course Conclusion

Get fresh and keep it fresh. Have sex in the kitchen, in the shower, with the lights on, in candlelight, in the car, in front of your video camera (and send us the tape), on a mountaintop, or break up the ritual and have a quickie. Be daring and get kinky.

Remember to vary your positions and rhythms, stay connected to your partner, talk to her, encourage her, tell her how great her pussy feels around your dick, and check in. The more you let her control the action, the more her pleasure will increase. That could mean that she tells you to get on top of her and fuck her, but at least she made the request. Be sure to learn all you can about how she likes to get stimulated during intercourse, and then follow through with some action. And when the intercourse is over, remember, the sex shouldn't be, unless you are *both* finished.

☀ Ass-istance for Two

Time to discuss that sweet erogenous zone we've all got down under—our anus. No one has a corner on anal pleasure. It's for lesbians, gay men, and heterosexuals alike. We even heard from some lesbians who actually entertain fantasies of turning over a boy! Maybe you'll do your lover, but maybe she might do you. We encourage you to consider embracing those fluid lesbian roles when it comes to this orifice.

The Big Taboo

Except for a perfunctory porno plunge, the anus is one of the great unexplored galaxies in the heterosexual world. This little love hole is surrounded by cultural taboos of homosexuality, deviance, and uncleanness. Yet for many people, the taboos around the anus are part of what make anal sex so much fun! For many who have made the initial expedition and never taken the trip again, the main inhibitor is pain. The initial pain and discomfort that come with anal sex is a natural event. For many women, their first experience with vaginal sex was surrounded by some pain or discomfort as well.

Men, this is a piece of information to hold on to and share with your lover when you talk to her about anal sex. Don't feel bad if the first time isn't astounding. First times are always hard. The first time a woman gives a blow job, her jaw might hurt or get sore, and your love rod might have received more teeth than you liked. There is a learning curve to everything. With respect to asses, this section is about getting you over the hump, so to speak.

> *I've explored anal pleasure with fingers only. I like it—it can help make an orgasm last and last. Its forbidden nature is what is erotic, I think.* —Curtis, 41, New York

Ass Comfort

All right, let's talk ass comfort. Most of our hesitations and judgments about the anus as a sexual pleasure zone have to do with our discomfort with our asses. Yeah, yeah, we've heard it all, "It's an exit, not an entrance." Let's put those clichés away for a bit. Funkadelic said it best: "Free your mind, and your ass will follow."

A lot of men and women are turned on by the idea of anal sex precisely because it is taboo. Anal-sex videos are their own cottage industry. Many men say they'd like to try it but would *never* initiate it with a partner—she would have to be the initiator. That is understandable, and since consent is necessary, it's a good policy. It's a hard subject to broach when you aren't sure if your partner will go for it. Be a rebel. Toss it in your phone sex or hot talk and see how she reacts. Then inquire within. Maybe your lover has been secretly wanting to try it too.

Our comfort with our asses has a lot to do with our comfort with poop. Face it, when dealing with assholes, you are going to deal with poop. It does live there. Most liaisons with the ass may be pretty low maintenance and no messes. But having some extra sex towels around is always a good idea, just in case.

⚡♡⚡ Honey, Come Closer

Anal play does not have to be an all-or-nothing proposition. It's not a choice between sticking a finger, penis, or toy up your lover's butt or completely avoiding the area altogether. You can lovingly explore its surface with kisses, licks, and massage strokes and see where that leads you.

Anal Starter Kit

Before you start, there are a few items you want on hand: a towel, a water-soluble lube, dental dams, latex gloves, and a washcloth or baby wipes (they can be convenient and fun, and they come with aloe vera and vitamin E).

Getting Going: Anal Sphincter Massage

Before you zero in on her butt, warm up the rest of her body. You know how to do that . . . kiss her and touch her all over just the way she likes it.

> *I tell my partner to sneak up on my asshole after lots of body love.*   —Shauna, 28, Minneapolis

When you begin to work on the sphincter, it's good for everyone to have a ritualistic cleansing. It's not uncommon to have a little fecal matter around the anus, no matter how diligently we try to wipe. So lovingly clean her with a damp cloth or one of the baby wipes. This will help put her at ease. She won't be nervously wondering the whole time whether her butt is clean. Now she will be free to enjoy the action. Better yet, you could take a bath or shower together. This could help you both relax.

One more time: Real life is not like porno. You can't just stick it in. Remember, this area is made up of muscles, and if they're tense, any penetration will hurt.

> *I have explored anal pleasure. It's a much more sensitive area to penetrate as far as the need to approach with care. I'm usually not relaxed enough to be comfortable.*
> —Jen, 25, New York

Start out by massaging her sphincter and the surrounding area, especially her perineum, an often neglected feel-good zone. Remember, that's the spot between the vulva and anus in women, and between the testicles and anus in men. You can use a little massage oil (use only a little) to make it easier. Connect with her in other ways while you massage to ease her vulnerability. Lay alongside her, your face in her ear, talking and kissing her sweetly.

As you massage her, ask her to take in deep breaths and relax. Ask her how the muscles feel. "Are they still tense or can you feel them relaxing?" If they are still tense, keep massaging and talking to your lover in a soft voice, encouraging her to relax, making her laugh.

Analingus

After massaging the whole anal area, some butt-lickin' fun might be in order. Analingus is a great pleasure for both men and women. Treat it gently, like you do her vulva. Those dental dams will come in handy. Slowly swirl your tongue around her anus. Feel all the little puckering skin around the hole—follow it, moving your tongue around it. The anus is highly sensitive, and your tongue will feel soothing. She may get very aroused from this, and if she relaxes, her anus will be ready for some introductory penetration.

> *What's not to like about rimming? The ass is a very sensitive place, and a soft tongue on it is a highly pleasurable thing! It relaxes my ass a lot, and it gets me really turned on. A little tongue fucking is quite nice too. I also like to give it because I know the pleasure it brings. I am into hygiene, though, so the ass needs to be clean for me to really feel comfortable and get into it.*   —Lynn, 25, Denver

It helps to prop her up with a pillow for easy access. She might need to get on all fours. The shower is an excellent place for analingus, because the hot water is relaxing and cleansing. While she stands with legs out, you can kneel down, spread her cheeks so you can get in there, and lick away.

If you're really daring, you can penetrate her anus with your tongue. Some thrusting in and out coupled with licking the rim—thus the term "rimming"—could feel mighty fine. Remember what you learned in the cunnilingus section about latex barriers? Revisit how to make your own dam out of a latex glove—it comes in handy for analingus as well. Lining her anus with the glove's little thumb will protect you from picking up an STI, and if you are one who is into extra cleanliness, it will take care of that concern as well.

Going In

Once she's fully relaxed, you can start to probe with fingers. Start with just one. Keep it simple.

Go slow! Not slow for *you*, slow for someone who has someone's finger up their ass. Ease the tip of your finger in, and linger a moment. Wait for the muscles to relax around your finger. As they do, you can push in a bit, then come almost all the way out. Then push in again, and out, then a little farther in again, slowly working your way in farther and farther, communicating with your partner all the way—"Is this good?" "Do you want me to stay inside, or go in and out a bit?" Also pay attention to the curve of her anus. It's not a straight shot, so have patience and find an angle that works. If it's uncomfortable for her, try other positions until it feels right.

The reaction of her body will tell you the most. If she's moaning and spreading her legs open farther and her anal sphincter muscles are relaxing, then you are on the right path. Keep it up. If she's tightening up and squirming, you want to check in to see if she's okay with the activity. Note: If you sense that something is wrong, don't just pull out all of a sudden—that can add to her discomfort or may not be what she wants. Warn her if you are going to pull out.

☼♡☼ Honey, Come Closer

When you first play with her anus, do it while licking her clit or sucking on nipples, especially if it's a new thing for her. If all the attention is on her ass, her anticipation of penetration may make her tense up. Pleasuring another surefire spot can help avoid this and facilitate a smooth ride in.

Lube It!

Okay, let's break this down. We've already discussed how unpleasant it is to have a dry clit stimulated. Doubly so for butt holes. There is no forgiveness in heaven for penetrating a dry asshole. Our anuses do not lubricate themselves the way vaginas do (and even there, a good lover will make sure to have plenty of lubrication before going in). The friction alone will leave your lover's butt chafed, red, and sore. Not fun.

If you have not yet acquainted yourself with the wonderful world of lube and you're wanting to experiment with some ass play, get yourself down to the nearest sex shop and pick up a variety pack! Water-based lubricant is a staple for any bedside table. You must lube *anything* that will go in her ass! Saliva can work, but it tends to dry up pretty fast, so adding some other lubricant is best.

Not all lube is created equal. We suggest a variety pack because you may want to try out different ones to see which work best for you and your partners. Some are stickier than others, some dry up faster, some feel oily, some have a consistency closer to natural human fluids. Once you find a lubricant you really like, get a big bottle of it and keep it handy. Our anuses are made of highly sensitive tissue and need to be treated with care. Anal penetration is only consistently painful when folks don't know what they are doing or don't take their time.

Safety

As with any sexual act where we are sharing bodily fluids and juicy parts, safety should be of the utmost concern. With anal play, there are some specific things to be aware of. When dealing with feces, you are dealing with bacteria. You want to be careful with that for a couple of reasons. In addition to other STIs, hepatitis A and hepatitis E can be transmitted sexually and through feces if you are with a partner who is infected. Also, if any residue from the anus gets into the vagina, your partner will get a yeast infection with a bite!

Lesbians are more sensitive to the issue of yeast infections because most have had one at some point. Women get them for a variety of reasons. It is not considered a sexually transmitted infection per se, but women can pass them to other women through sex.

> ### ☼♡☼ Honey, Come Closer
>
> *Never, ever* put anything that has been in her ass (or yours—or anywhere else, for that matter) in or near her vagina. This is *extremely* important. It will completely disrupt her natural yeast balance, an infection will follow closely thereafter, and you will get NO pussy for a very long time. You don't want that. She will not be a happy camper, and it certainly could put a damper on any future excursions with the anus.

Lesbians are also familiar with the notion of latex gloves, and using them during anal play is a good idea. You have to remember which finger has been where and be sure to use the right one in the right orifice. A good way to go is to designate a hand for each orifice if you are ambidextrous enough. Your left hand can be for ass and your right hand for pussy, or vice versa. Still, it's easy to mix them up, so using a glove for any anal contact is a good idea, because afterward you can just take it off and use your hands freely.

Another excellent little latex device is finger cots—little condoms for fingers. They are particularly good for anuses, especially if she's only into one or two fingers. They're easy and not messy. You simply roll 'em on and roll 'em off when you're through. They are often distributed in safer-sex packets and should also be available in doctors' offices, good drugstores, or medical-supply stores.

Remember: Never use any type of oil with latex. Oil destroys latex. This means big holes in condoms or gloves—not a road you want to wander down naively. Oil-based lubes include Vaseline, baby oil, massage oil, cooking oils, Crisco, or anything else that contains oil. Some people like oil-based lubes for anal play because of their slickness, but for safety, it's always best to use a water-based lubricant with condoms.

Why Go Anal?

Being penetrated makes us vulnerable and opens us up. When penetrated anally, we open up our root chakras and our bodies in a profound way. We carry a lot of tension in our ass. Allowing it to be penetrated releases a lot of that tension and can relax us, but we *have* to be relaxed enough to even try. Once we do, our energy begins to flow in a very different way with anal penetration.

> *I think the world would be a better place if everyone could open up and allow themselves to be penetrated in their asses . . . it's taboo: it's that deep, dark place that you aren't supposed to talk about, touch, or sexualize. It goes beyond sexualizing it . . . it opens us up physically, spiritually, and emotionally. For some, that's too much to handle. I love the intensity.*   —Jackie, 38, Santa Barbara, California

Women who have had positive experiences with anal penetration speak to how it differs from vaginal penetration. Some attest that the orgasms they have when anal penetration is involved (usually coupled with clitoral and/or vaginal stimulation) are far more powerful than other orgasms. For those of you who haven't tried it, maybe it's time to get over your anal phobia and let the play begin.

> *My orgasms have been incredibly enhanced by anal stimulation. I've never had an orgasm from anal play alone. But one that comes with anal and clitoral stimulation is much more intense than a purely clitoral orgasm.*
> —Suzanne, 29, New York

I come so much harder when my butt is being fingered too.
—Donna, 22, Jersey City, New Jersey

Anal Slow Dancing with Your Penis

So maybe you've experimented with fingers for a while and you and your partner have decided to go for broke and try anal intercourse. You know the basics: lots of building up, lots of relaxation, lots of lube. Okay, now you're ready to penetrate. Use all your new lesbian skills. Stay in communication as you work the head of your cock in. Help her relax with soothing talk, kisses, and gentle caresses with your hands and fingers on her breasts and vulva.

As with vaginal penetration, you don't want to just stick your whole lubed dick in all at once. Take it slow, as you did with your fingers. Once the head is in, pull out a bit, then ease in a little more. Keep pushing in a little more each time, with long pauses so her anus can adjust to the sensation. Make sure she'll tell you if anything hurts. Add more lube as needed.

> *I find I have to use lots of lube and water and a vibrator to stimulate my clit because anal penetration is a different and sometimes more intense experience. I need the clit stimulation to aid at the beginning of penetration. Once the object of choice has fully entered my anus, the humping and bumping can begin with or without the clitoral stimulation. I have also found that the more control I have of entry, the better. I like to be on top of the person or object for the beginning.*
> —Jillian, 26, Brooklyn

Once you're in and she's comfortable, you can slowly start to move. As with your first attempts at vaginal intercourse (if you're an anal virgin or close to it), you are venturing into a whole new world. You and your lover will have to explore and experiment to find your anal style. How does she like you to move? Deep or shallow? Slow and easy or fast and hard? You'll also need to explore different positions: her on top, you on top, from behind, standing up with her lying on a bed or high piece of furniture.

Which positions are best for stimulating her clitoris, for inserting a dildo into her vagina, or both? This is a great time to introduce a vibrator. Since you both will have a lot to concentrate on, the vibe can take care of her clit, bringing her pleasure and keeping her relaxed. Let the pleasure begin.

Roll Over!

The best advice for men is that they should really learn to be comfortable and open to being penetrated anally. I think anal penetration for men is especially important because I do think the G-spot for men is at the base of their spine, and so anal penetration really does stimulate this part more directly. And to think the poor straight men have been denying themselves really intense orgasms because they feel like they have to uphold the image of always being the "top" or the "penetrator" since this is supposed to be a "masculine" role—or else they never even thought that there could be other options in sex other than penile-vaginal intercourse!
—Sam, 34, Brooklyn

I turned a guy over and fucked him with my fingers. Probably one of the hottest sexual experiences in my life.
—Karen, 24, Queens, New York

Now for the big question: Have you ever thought about letting your girlfriend roll you over and do you up the butt? Many women fantasize about doing this to their male partners. They long to feel what it's like to "be on the other side," to possess another kind of power within sex, and to have their male partner get in touch with what it's like to be penetrated.

I would love to [put on a strap-on and turn him over], but my boyfriend won't let me. What is it about that that makes men so afraid? It's so stigmatized as a "gay" thing that it's like they question their own sexuality if their cheeks are

*opened. It's only lately that my boyfriend will even let me
touch his ass.* —Melynda, 22, Holland

Consider this: How can you justify penetrating partners over and over when you have never been penetrated yourself? If you are firmly against letting your partners touch your ass, ask yourself why. If it's because you'll go through some kind of identity crisis or think you'll be perceived as gay, then get over it! Gay folk don't have a lock on anal pleasure. It seems clear that homophobia is the number one reason why straight men do not explore their asses. A little anal indulgence does not mean you will be hanging out at the local gay bar and that your whole identity will come into question. Please consider your poor, neglected ass for a minute. You might be surprised how sweet it can be. Granted, it may not be for everyone, but don't knock it till you give it a few tries.

*He liked me to use a dildo while I was giving him a blow
job. It relaxed him a lot, and he had an awesome orgasm.
I enjoyed being able to offer him something different.*
—Juanita, 26, San Antonio

Men, your anus can be a whole new zone to play with! Having another playground to make whoopie on takes pressure off your penis.

☼♡ Honey, Come Closer

Many men say that their orgasms are much more powerful when their anus is involved. You have something in your anus that the ladies don't: the prostate gland. This is a well-known pleasure spot for men. Often referred to as the "male G-spot," it likes to be stimulated. They way to reach it is . . . yep, you guessed it, through your butt hole.

Your prostate is located just below the bladder. It's about the size of a walnut in a young man, and it gets larger as you age.

> *I have never had an actual orgasm from strictly anal play, but when the penis is also involved, it can be a positively delightful combination.*   —Richard, 50, Berkeley, California

Everything we've just talked about regarding anuses goes for yours too. Move slow, relax it, start small, and work up. If you decide you only want to stay with external touching or the little finger, that's fine. But if you are daring, there is a good chance you will have a partner who would love to turn you over and do you. Give it up and enjoy the ride.

If you're having a lot of trouble with this whole concept, you may be having a hard time letting go of the roles you are used to playing. This is an area where lesbians are often at a great advantage. Their roles are not so rigidly defined, and they can create whatever dynamics they want to within sexual relationships. This is very freeing and allows for experimentation, expansion, and evolution in the way sex is experienced. If you learn anything from this book, learn this. Let go of any rigidity you are hanging on to for dear life, and allow yourself to go to new places sexually and sensually. Have sex as a means of enjoying the ride, *wherever* it takes you, instead of driving toward one specific destination all the time. That ride gets boring in a hurry. You can surrender to the journey whether you are into anal play or not. Find your own ways to let go and seek new levels. They are there, and you will find them through open communication and a willing partner.

Expanding
the
Horizons

☀ Boys and Their Toys

I am in a relationship of almost eight years. We both LOVE sex-toy sex; it has enhanced our sex life as a couple tremendously. If it's late and we're tired but in the mood, vibrators jazz up our sexual energy and arousal levels IMMEDIATELY! We've come up with all kinds of vibrator positions, from enhancing full-body, "look ma, no hands" contact, to complete visual access.
— Robyn, 40, Brooklyn

Toy Joy

Although sex toys date back to before recorded time, they are still shrouded in misunderstanding, misconception, and negative connotations. They're still hidden under the bed, in drawers, and in closets. Whatever people think about sex toys they may also think about the people who use them.

Lesbians are no strangers to sex toys. Some people may think their heavy use of toys shows that they are sexually unfulfilled in other ways or need help. Actually, we can attribute the popularity of toys among lesbians to their fluid roles and wide spectrum of possibilities in the pursuit of sexual pleasure. Lesbians know pleasure comes in a whole array of packages, which on one day might be sensuous kissing and manual stimulation of genitals, and on another, a wild, acrobatic fucking session with a strap-on coupled with a vibrator for the clitorises!

We have very open minds and talk about things we like. A few years ago we decided to get a vibrator and both enjoyed the newness.   —Christie, 26, Central, Pennsylvania

We encountered a range of responses about toys. Many people told stories of how toys enhance their sex lives. Others weren't as open. One man said, "I don't need the help," reinforcing the idea that the only people who use sex toys are those who can't manage their pleasure on their own. Whatever your preconceived ideas about sex toys, open your mind for a bit and listen to what toys represent in the lesbian bedroom. You may be surprised.

Not all lesbians like toys. But I think toys are great! I think of them as things to assist in play. They can be as simple as a dildo, a vibrator, or they can be different costumes. If you let go they can assist in the sensations or feelings. If you are with a girl who wants clitoral stimulation it can be so nice to have a vibrator there to help out while you're doing other things. You have to give yourself time to get used to things, but it's what you make of it.   —Patricia, 35, Arlington, Virginia

Vibrators: Not Just for Ladies

Vibrators were invented in the late nineteenth century by American doctors to treat women diagnosed with "female disorders." They were used for genital massage, a standard medical practice, to induce "hysterical paroxysm" (orgasm) in patients. If vibrators could win the Nobel Peace Prize, we might award it for helping to create self-love by the millions.

My boyfriend should love my vibrator. It satisfies me at a pure sexual level so I don't go guy crazy when he's not around.   —Karen, 29, Tempe, Arizona

Vibrators are a familiar friend to the lesbian tribe. In general, they are more popular among women, although many men also enjoy the intense stimulation of a vibrator. You can use one along your shaft, around your testicles, on your perineum, around the anus, inside the anus, to stimulate your prostate, and on your nipples. There are many vibrators made especially for men that can be worn around the testicles and/or at the base of the penis.

Reasons to Consider Adding a Vibrator to Your Toybox

- To break the monotony and spice up sex. Different types of stimulation can provide different kinds of orgasms and pleasure.
- They provide consistently strong stimulation for both men and women. Women, in particular, often require consistent and intense stimulation that vibrators provide quite well. Bonus—no hand cramps!
- For pre-orgasmic women, vibrators are an invaluable tool for learning how to reach orgasm.
- They give extra pleasure during sex, possibly freeing hands for other things (depending on the type of vibrator).
- They can be used all over the body, and you may discover new erotic zones you didn't know you had.
- You and a partner can use a vibrator simultaneously and share the vibes.
- It means your penis doesn't always have to be the star.

Sensitivity

For women who are not used to a vibrator, the stimulation can actually be too intense. That's okay. Not every woman will like the stimulation of some vibrators. But for many women, they provide a welcome enhancement of their pleasure. There is a range in the power and longevity of vibrators. It is possible to get one to provide more diffuse sensations, as well as one that provides more intense vibrations.

No Competition

A common fear some men have is that their lover will "get addicted" to her vibrator and won't need him anymore. A vibrator and a loving human being are two very different things. You will still be needed, appreciated, and enjoyed in any healthy relationship. You are her lover. A toy does not replace the eroticism of a live body and the emotional and psychological connection she hopefully has with you. A toy can only enhance that connection due to your openness to try it and experiment.

The stimulation a vibrator provides for a woman's clitoris is definitely different from your tongue, fingers, or other toys. There may be times when she would prefer one type over another. Women can get accustomed to vibrator stimulation, but the healthiest way to think about it is as something to incorporate to make it more fun.

> ### ⦂♡⦂ Honey, Come Closer
>
> Vibrators are not your competition, but a helpful addition.

Choosing a Vibrator

A vibrator is a wonderful gift to give your partner, and it can bring both of you additional pleasure no one will be complaining about. There are hundreds of different vibrators on the market. Consider the following things when choosing one.

Power. Vibrators can be plug-in, which provide consistently strong vibrations and tend to have a longer life span, or battery operated, which are inexpensive, portable, and offer gentle vibrations but may not last as long. Vibrators that use C batteries tend to be stronger than those that use AA batteries, so you want to decide how strong a vibrator you want to get. There is a wide range.

Speed. It may be important to you or your partner whether the vibrator is a variable-speed vibe, which can be adjusted specifically for a person's pleasure, or has limited speeds—usually two or three settings.

Price. The third thing to think about is how much you want to spend. Prices range from $10 for a novelty type that probably won't last very long, to $70, $80, even $100 for those on the high end. Keep in mind that a vibrator is an investment with many happy returns!

Adaptability. Some vibrators are made for penetration, and some are not. Some come with fancy attachments or have multifaceted capabilities. Think about what you want to be able to use your vibrator for before deciding what type to buy.

The First Lady of Vibrators

There is no one who singlehandedly did more to make vibrators a household word than the "Godmother of Masturbation" herself, Betty Dodson, who popularized a "back massager" called the Hitachi Magic Wand, now commonly known as the Cadillac of vibrators. For more than thirty years in her BodySex workshops and private coaching sessions, she has taught thousands of women about their genitals, how to love them and how to have orgasms. She has worked with couples and men as well, helping them to overcome sexual barriers and expand their erotic potential.

Dodson promotes the Hitachi because it is a plug-in wand vibrator that provides powerful vibes and has a long life span. Use it on the whole vulva, or the penis and testicles, as well as for sore necks and backs (which is how it is advertised and promoted, of course)! The head is soft and diffuses the strong vibrations, which can be too strong for some people. Sometimes the vibrations can be so intense that the nerves in the clitoris or penis may numb a bit temporarily. An easy way to remedy this is by using a towel as a buffer between the genitals and the vibrator to avoid "numbing out." You can, for instance, start with two or four layers of a towel or cloth and work down to one or none, depending on your preference.

Wand-type vibrators are not made for penetration, but there are attachments available that can be used for insertion in the vagina or anus. Attachments can distribute vibrations better or spread them out more evenly. They also may diffuse particularly strong vibrations. Examples are *come cups* for men, which fit around the head of the penis, or a *G-spotter,* which has a curved angle and fits over a wand. Because of the G-spotter's angle, it can be used for penetration in women to stimulate the urethral sponge (G-spot) and, in men, to stimulate the prostate gland anally. Double the pleasure!

Shopping

Some vibrators are quite simple, while others are pretty fancy with a price tag to match. Some women like penetration with a vibrating toy in their vagina or anus. There are vibrators that come with multiple functions and gauges for each, like a rotating phallus, with bunny ears up top for her clitoris. Both parts vibrate simultaneously. The rotation may also stimulate the G-spot. If either you or your partner want a vibrator for insertion in your anus, be sure it has a flared base, because a small one all lubed up could easily slip into your rectum and be difficult to remove. You wouldn't want to find yourself in the emergency room unexpectedly!

Questions to ask yourself when choosing a vibrator:

- Will sound bother me? (Some vibrators are louder than others.) Be sure to check it out before you buy.
- How powerful do I want my vibrations?
- Do I want something portable?
- Do I want a vibrator that can be used for penetration of the anus or vagina?
- Do I want variable speed, or are one or two settings okay?
- How much do I want to spend?

Go shopping and have some fun. You can either give it as a surprise gift to your lover or go shopping with her and pick something out together. If you go to a reputable sex-toy store, the clerks are usually pretty helpful and knowledgeable. Don't be shy. Go in and ask lots of questions.

Rookies and Pros: Getting to Know Your Power Tools

The best way to get to know her vibrator is to play with it yourself. Okay, get a firm grasp and turn the vibrator on, first on low, then through the various speeds. Feel the difference in intensity of each level. Hold it against your belly and feel the way the vibrations travel down to your groin. Move it up the length of your torso; tease it over one nipple, then the other. What does it feel like? Good? Too intense? Do you like lighter stimulation, or do you prefer the powerful sensation of deep pressure at full throttle?

These are the variations in sensation that you'll be applying to your lover's body, and you want to be as sensitive to her as you are to your own reactions. Run the vibrator back down your torso to the base of your cock and tease around it without actually touching the shaft. Run down your inner thigh, under your scrotum, and feel the sensation of both light and deep vibration on your perineum, the sensitive place above your anus and below your balls.

Run it down to the outside of your anus, not entering, just teasing, and feel how those vibrations shoot all through your pelvis without any penetration at all. Play with whisper-soft touches, firm touches, and deep, grinding vibrations that rock through you.

Remember, all of this is on the outside of your big, masculine body. Now, imagine these same sensations on the incredibly sensitive exposed clitoris, or thrusting inside of the delicate membranes of her sweet vagina. Makes you realize what a deft touch a vibrator requires, doesn't it? The great thing about using a vibrator on your lover is that your brain is not lodged inside your cock, at least not like it is when you're fucking her. You can pay more attention to her and really learn her body's cues and signals so that the next time you penetrate her with your own warm self, you'll be an even better lover.

Word to the wise, guys: You can fry a clit with too much vibratory pressure—that is, temporarily desensitize your lover instead of bringing her to orgasm. But with thoughtful, indeed artful use, the vibrator can be an amazing enhancer of sex.

:♡: **Honey, Come Closer**

If your lover already owns a vibrator, ask her to show you how she uses it. Then use it on her and incorporate it into your lovemaking as she likes.

For those who are new to this toy, here's a little blueprint. Make her feel nice and relaxed first. Start by giving her lots of kisses, then use the vibrator on her neck, shoulders, and upper chest. Let the larger muscles of her body get used to the sensations. Be careful around bony areas. Then move down to her thighs, the outside first, then moving to her inner thighs, working your way slowly to her vulva. Move the vibrator over her belly and to her breasts and use it to stimulate her nipples. Then go back down to the inner thighs and this time start to stimulate her outer lips with light buzzes, then her pubic mound, sending vibrations through her clitoris. Then explore the inner lips and her vaginal opening, but don't penetrate—not yet. Go down and give her clit some yummy kisses and a little sucking so it's aroused and swollen. Finally, go to town on her clit, stimulating the shaft, hood, and glans if she can take it. If you are using a vibrator made for penetration, you might explore some in-and-out vibe love with her pussy. Find her favorite spots. You can ask her to use it on herself the way she likes it while you play with the rest of her body, and as always, take avid notes!

:♡: **Honey, Come Closer**

Many women report having much stronger orgasms with simultaneous vaginal penetration and clitoral stimulation. You can stimulate her clitoris with the vibrator while penetrating her vagina with your finger. Another option, especially if you'd like to get your penis involved, is to use a vibe on her clit while having intercourse. This is one of the best ways to insure that your partner has an orgasm during vaginal penetration.

Safety and Cleaning

- The best way to prevent passing on sexually transmitted infections through toys is not to share yours with others—each partner uses only his or her own goods.
- Many vibrators can be used with condoms. If you are sharing with a partner, be sure to use a new condom over it when the toy changes hands. You can even get a condom over the Hitachi head. You can also use two condoms and take one off for the next partner or for another orifice.
- You should clean your toys after each use so bacteria doesn't grow on them. If you are allergic to latex or don't want to use condoms for some other reason, you should always clean toys after one person uses them before they are used on another.
- You can clean toys with any germicidal cleanser, such as rubbing alcohol or hydrogen peroxide, or with special cleansers that are sold in any sex-toy shop (but tend to be more expensive than the more easily accessible household items). You can also use soap and water, and that should suffice.
- Vibrators shouldn't be immersed in water—you never want to immerse a plug-in vibe! They can be wiped clean with a cloth moistened with warm water and antibacterial soap, then again with plain water to get rid of the cleaning-agent residue. Vinyl vibrator attachments like the Hitachi G-spotter can even be washed in the top rack of a dishwasher.

Dildos and Harnesses

Dildos are nonvibrating toys used by both men and women for penetration of the vagina, anus, or mouth. They create a sensation of fullness and pressure that many people find highly pleasurable. They can be held in the hand or strapped on using a harness. Although the world "dildo" comes from the Italian word *diletto*, meaning "delight," dildos probably carry more stigma and misconception than any other sex toy, especially regarding lesbians' use of them.

Harnesses, a.k.a. strap-ons, hold the dildo and attach it to the body against the pubic bone by wrapping around the waist and pelvis. There are harnesses that are worn around the thigh as well. If you want to wear a dildo in a harness, you will need a dildo with a wide or flared base so it won't slip out.

Having Everything

Some of the men in our groups expressed confusion about why a lesbian would need to use a dildo. "Isn't that just imitating a man?" One lesbian responded poignantly, "No. It's getting the best of both worlds. I can have a female partner and all the benefits of her female body—her soft skin and breasts—and she can penetrate me with her own cock. She has breasts *and* a dick."

For lesbians who enjoy penetration, a woman with a phallus is a very good thing. It doesn't mean she's trying to imitate a man or a heterosexual relationship. Quite the contrary: A woman who know how to wield her dick is as queer as it gets! A woman who straps on a dildo and fucks her partner is totally different from a man utilizing his penis. Still, there is a whole range of feelings within the lesbian community about strap-ons. Some lesbians don't see them as a positive thing but as contradictory to lesbian sexual culture. Many lesbians would never use one.

Lesbian Cocks

Many women feel an emotional and psychological connection to their cock. It is not just an artificial appendage for many. Some lesbians identify as "butch" or even as "boys," and their cock is linked to their masculinized identity. This does not mean they are "trying to be men." If we look at gender in a more fluid way, we can recognize that there is a wide range of female experiences and an equally large range of male experiences. A butch woman is not a man. She is in her own gender category. Many women are erotically attracted to butches but would never go near a genetic man. People express their gender in different ways, and it is too simplistic to think we all fall into one of two categories.

> *We use dildos with harness when we know we have pro-longed time for sex and can really savor it. It's a turn-on to "pack" in public and surprise my partner by rubbing up against her.* —Jenna, 39, Seattle

It's not just the butches who love their dildos. They are worn and enjoyed by all kinds of women. And not all women connect to their dildos psychologically. They can be simply another tool for pleasure.

One woman explained in one of our groups that part of her joy in using her strap-on is that the base of her dildo sits against her clitoris, so with the motion of the fucking, her clit gets stimulated. While penetrating a partner she can have orgasms. All of the men were amazed at this, never having connected how a strap-on might assist in physical pleasure for the person wearing it, not to mention all of the psychological components that are a big part of the turn-on.

> *I used to always have to strap it on and when I did, it auto-matically became my cock so it could feel like an extension of me. But now I feel like all my toys are an extension of me whether they're on my body or not. I don't have to strap it on to feel like that.* —Lynn, 29, Pittsburgh

Why You Should Own at Least One Dildo

- Dildos are not penis substitutes—they provide variety and options for our changing sexual appetites.
- Many men and women enjoy penetration, and each person has different preferences for length and width of penetrative objects. Dildos allow us to customize the size we want.
- With dildos, we can have penetration any time—not only

when we have an aroused and willing male partner. Many people like to use them when they masturbate.

- Some women like simultaneous penetration of the vagina and the anus.
- For folks interested in anal sex, dildos are useful since you can start small and work up to larger sizes as your rectum expands. Remember that rectums and anuses are sensitive and require patience and care.
- Dildos can be helpful for women or men who want to experiment with penetration without the added anxiety of a partner being present, or help when a partner is present to demonstrate what you like.
- They can be a helpful way to practice performing fellatio before trying it on an actual partner.
- They are great for men who want to be penetrated by a female partner. She can wear it or use it manually.

Men and Dildos

I haven't strapped it on and done him yet, but I have one. I'm just waiting for him to give in. He penetrates himself alone. I think he's scared for me to do it.
                                    —Sandra, 24, Los Angeles

Some men's discomfort with dildos may be linked to what dildos represent to them. The phallus has traditionally been a physical representation of male power and privilege, so it may be threatening to some men to see that women can handle that kind of power too. It could also be a turn-on. Many men's discomfort about dildos, especially if they are to be worn by their partner, is connected to their own homophobia. Please remember that a person's sexual identity is very different from the sexual behaviors he or she likes or does.

> ### ⟡ Honey, Come Closer
>
> Don't think that because you have a penis you are beyond dildo use. In fact, there are many excellent reasons for using dildos, and you may find them to be an exciting addition to your sexual practices, as well.

Why Would a Man Want to Use a Strap-on?

I occasionally use a dildo on myself or my partner. It depends entirely on the partner. My latest partner was not into it at all. I would like a partner who wants to use a vibrator or other sex toys during sex, simply as part of being uninhibited and trying new things. —Gary, 41, Boston

It takes quite a man to be willing to don a dildo. For men with open minds, there are many good reasons to consider using a strap-on. First of all, it can be a lot of fun. You can fantasize about being a two-dicked man for double the pleasure, double the fun. If you have a partner who likes to be penetrated in her anus and her vagina simultaneously, there are ways to manipulate your penis and a strap-on to provide a "double fuck." Dildos also provide variety in size, which may be important to your partner. You can use a strap-on when you are without erection for any reason.

Also, for men with physical disabilities, dildos can restore their ability to please a partner with a phallus, opening up sexual possibility and likely giving them a boost in sexual self-esteem. In fact, one major manufacturer of high-quality dildos was started by a disabled man.

And let's not forget that many heterosexual men enjoy being penetrated anally. Your partner can strap one on and fuck you, which not only feels good but can be a fun role-reversal and a great way to expand your sexual pleasure. Many women fantasize about what it would be like to be the "fucker." This is a great way for her to show you how she would like you to fuck *her*.

> ### ☼ Honey, Come Closer
>
> If you ejaculate and lose your erection but your partner wants to keep fucking, you can prolong the session by using a dildo. In doing so, you are showing sensitivity for your partner's needs, rather than focusing the fucking around you and your penis's timeline of pleasure—a big complaint of heterosexual women.

Choosing and Using a Dildo

Dildos come in various widths, lengths, shapes, colors, and styles, so you can get one customized with all the qualities you are looking for. Some are "penislike," textured with veins and all, and some take on the less realistic shapes of animals or art deco designs. There are stylized, art-object-type dildos, made from wood, hard plastic, ceramic, leather, chrome, lucite, or acrylic. Most typically, dildos are made of silicone, which is resilient, retains body heat, and is easy to clean; or rubber, which is soft, porous, and not as easy to clean (it's best to use condoms with them). Some dildos come with a nifty little curve, which can be helpful in stimulating the G-spot in women or the prostate gland in men. And remember, if you plan to use a dildo in a harness, it must have a flared base. Some have other features, like a removable suction cup at the base so that it can be attached to a hard surface for straddling during solo play.

> *A lot of my partners have enjoyed being penetrated in both their pussy and their ass at the same time. It's much easier to be able to sit and manually do it with both hands. Sometimes there's not enough room to have my body up against her. I can control it better and it looks good.*
>
> —Barbara, 32, Chicago

You also need to figure out how wide and how long a dildo you or your partner want. For vaginal penetration, this largely depends on whether women like deeper penetration that may hit the cervix or more shallow penetration. For anal insertion, both men and women may want to start small and work up to larger dildos, unless you have had larger items in your anus before. Dildos aren't exchangeable, so make sure your eyes aren't bigger than your orifice! Don't forget that if you are planning to use your dildo with a harness, you will lose at least a half inch off its length during use.

ༀ Honey, Come Closer

As with vibrators, get to know your dildo. If you're planning on sticking it up her butt, you should know what it feels like up yours.

Harness Up

Harnesses are generally made out of either fabric, nylon, or leather. Fabric harnesses are machine washable and economical, while leather ones are more comfortable, durable, and expensive. Leather harnesses have a longer life span, so they are good if you think you will be into this practice; if you entertain a leather fetish, there's a bonus. The harness has a ring that holds the dildo in. Metal rings may be appealing to some folks, but the more flexible latex rings are better for your dildos.

Harnesses come in a few styles. The two-strap type can be used by both men and women, and fits men most comfortably. The straps wrap around each leg, allowing more access to the anus and genitals of the wearer. Two-straps tend to be more stable and less wobbly and also fit larger people better. A single-strap harness can be worn as a cock ring for men and used by women. Anyone who doesn't like wearing a thong or g-string will not like this type, because the strap runs between the butt cheeks. On the other hand, some may like the stimulation of a strap between their buttocks. There are harnesses that attach the dildo to a person's thigh for a different variation.

Make sure the ring size on the harness is big enough to accommodate all of the dildos you may want to use with it. If you think you will be using a wide variety of sizes, you might want a harness with snaps for changing the ring size. Again, harnesses aren't necessarily cheap. You may want to start with a cheaper fabric harness if you are unsure of how much you will get into harness play. If you are more serious, a more expensive leather harness is a better buy in the long run.

Safety and Cleaning

- Once again, lubricant is very important, as dildos do not self-lubricate like genitals. Some rubber dildos are porous and will soak up juices. Be sure to lube up the dildo as well as the orifice it will be used in, unless it is to be used in a mouth, in which case lube is not necessary and probably wouldn't be real tasty (unless you have some flavored lube you like!).
- Always wash dildos thoroughly after use with warm water and antibacterial soap or a special sex-toy cleaning agent, and rinse well. If they get dust and other particles on them in between use, you may want to wash them right before the next use. Even better—store dildos in their own dust-free plastic bag.
- You can also boil silicone dildos in a saucepan on the stove for three minutes to sterilize them. Do not boil rubber dildos, because they won't look like dildos when you're finished!
- After washing dildos, it's best to let them air dry before putting them away, as towels contain dust and lint particles that will attach themselves to the dildo. Viruses and bacteria won't live on a dry surface. To maintain its shape, store your dildo upright.
- If you and your partner share a dildo, do so with caution. Either use it with a condom that's changed before you switch off, or use two and remove one for the second partner. Or wash the dildo thoroughly before using it on the next person to avoid exchange of bodily fluids.
- It is recommended that you *always use condoms with rubber dildos* because they are more porous and therefore

more difficult to clean. Tacky, porous surfaces are an ideal place for bacteria to grow. Using condoms can also add years to the life of a cheap rubber dildo.

- Also, *never* put anything that has been in an anus into the vagina or mouth without cleaning or changing condoms, as it will cause a painful bacterial infection. The best way to avoid problems is, again, to use condoms for each orifice, or take the condom off when you are finished with anal play, so the dildo is bacteria-free for the vagina.
- Harnesses can be wiped down with cleanser on a damp cloth, then wiped clean. You can buy special leather oils to keep leather harnesses soft.

Why You and Your lover Should Consider Strapping It On

- For both men and women who want penetration that is risk free, strap-ons are a great way to go.
- For women interested in gender play, dildos are a great asset for exploring their male personas or the boy within. For many women, donning a phallus can be the ultimate gender bender. Some women like to be women with a penis! When first trying one on, a woman may feel anything from ridiculous to powerful.
- Strap-ons can create a radical role switch during sex and open up your repertoire of fantasy and role-play.
- Men can wear dildos too, either for the erotic thrill of it, or if they are without erection and their partner wants to be penetrated.
- For women who like double penetration of vagina and anus, a male partner can strap a dildo on and use it in one and his penis in the other. There are also ways women can strap on two dildos simultaneously for double penetration of a partner, or to have one for herself and one in her lover.
- Strap-ons free hands for other play.

Anal Toys

Now that you've been introduced to the joys of anal play, let's talk about some fun toys to give you some ass-istance.

Beads: New Ways to Accessorize

Anal beads are a popular toy to start off with because they are small. They are generally made of rubber or plastic strung on a nylon cord, and come in sizes ranging from marbles to softballs. Many people like the feel of the anus opening and closing around each bead. They can be fun to insert, one by one. Many people like to have the string pulled out at the moment of climax, as it increases their pleasure by intensifying the orgasmic contractions; for other folks, this may be too intense, so beads are better pulled out before or after orgasm. With plastic beads, use a nail file to smooth any sharp seams before you use them—we don't want any ass-aults.

Plug It In

Butt plugs come in a variety of shapes, sizes, and colors. They are similar to dildos in many ways, except that they are smaller and shaped a bit differently, including a flared base so they don't slip into the rectum. Many people like the full feeling of having a butt plug in their anus. Vibrating plugs can be pleasurable, but for some people they're uncomfortable and may make them feel like their bowels are moving. For those who like them, vibrating plugs are a flexible option because, depending on your mood, you can use them with or without the vibration.

Use a condom over a vibrating plug for the safest, easiest, least messy play. Some plugs are made out of jelly rubber and are more porous, so take the same precautions as you would for dildos so bacteria doesn't build up.

Relaxing the anal sphincter muscles is important for enjoyable anal play. A large exhale will make it easier to slide an anal plug or dildo in, and you might be tired of hearing it, but it bears

repeating: lube, lube, and more lube! The importance and ne-
cessity of lubricant for anal play cannot be underestimated. As
we've said, the anus does not lubricate itself, so have plenty of
lube on hand and use it generously. Because the anus is made
of pretty sensitive tissue, it requires care, as it can tear easily, but
it is possible to stretch it and work up to larger butt toys with
some practice and patience.

Other Toys

Nipple Clamps

Many men and women like the intense sensation of having
their nipples clamped. Clamps provide a piercing sensation, and
the longer you leave them on, the more intense it feels when
you remove them. After a while, the nipples numb a little, so
when you remove the clamps, they wake up! Nipple clamps are
popular for bondage, which we'll discuss in more depth later in
"What's the Kink?" Many men never think to explore their nipples, yet they can give much pleasure, so even if you're not into
the heightened sensations of clamps, don't forget your nipples.

ꙮ Honey, Come Closer

Since a toy can be any implement that enhances sexual pleasure, you can use your imagination to create
practically any sex toy you can dream up.

Make Your Own Device

Be inventive. Look around your house. Try a clean feather
duster for a full-body, sensuous turn-on; a kitchen spatula for a
hot, stinging spanking; a bandanna for a blindfold; or clothes-
pins for nipple clamps. You dream it and you can probably in-
vent it. Just have fun, explore, and be safe about it!

We take toys with us when we travel, which is exciting, because in that action alone we've made the commitment to have sex, even if we don't end up using them.
—Denise, 35, Springfield, Illinois

As we hope we've made clear, sex toys are not just chick stuff. Many toys are made especially for men. You may want to explore what's on the market for your pleasure as well as your lover's. Remember, toys are an enhancement that can add variety.

One heterosexual woman said she didn't need "props." Maybe sex toys can be thought of as props. What do props traditionally do? They help tell a story, they add to an environment, they enhance a scene. Not every scene needs a prop. But they can add a fun, light comic element or make for some intensely pleasurable drama. Great artists explore all the options.

☀ Hand Love

Hand love is the extension of all we discussed in "Finger Love: Becoming a Digital Master" back in the "Sapphic Arts" chapter. Hand love is commonly referred to as "vaginal fisting" because it involves carefully working a whole hand into the vagina and making a fist once inside. Because of that name, it often gets a bad rap as being something "violent" or scary. Quite the contrary. It is inarguably one of the most intimate, intense sexual acts happening in LesbianLand and requires trust, absolute desire, and know-how.

Hand Love Is Not for Everybody

You may not want to run out and try fisting after reading this section. It is definitely not for everyone. It's not even for all lesbians, though it's probably much more popular among Sapphic lovers. It is a practice to be approached with caution and respect. To be allowed to put one's hand inside a woman, to literally reach inside of her, is a great honor. It is also one of the most intimate ways you can possibly connect to her. You are totally linked— your arm in her pelvis, rocking, pushing in and out, tickling her womb, or being still. You are feeling every nook and cranny of her love canal while her heartbeat pulsates around your hand.

Hand love is not an everyday event but one for "special occasions." It takes a lot of time, patience, and trust. It's not kid stuff, and you *can* hurt her or yourself if you don't use caution or do it right. So respect it and follow the rules if you're going to add this to your sexual repertoire.

Size Matters

Some women have smaller pelvises than others, and this can determine whether or not she can take a whole hand inside her. Certainly a woman who does not like vaginal penetration or anything large in her vagina will not be a likely fisting candidate. However, for a woman who likes vaginal penetration, it can be exhilarating to share her most sacred space with a lover in this unique way.

> *I wasn't really sure why anyone would want my whole hand in there until I met someone who was big enough to accommodate, and who clearly enjoyed the experience. I certainly would advise caution when attempting it, starting with one finger and working up. Lots of lube is necessary. So are well-attended fingernails, and a lot of patience.*
> —Jack, 54, Chicago

The size of your hand is also a factor. This may be part of the reason fisting appears to be more popular between women than it is between men and women: Women's hands are generally smaller, and there are more potential pussies for a small-handed fister. The larger your hands, the slower you need to go. If you have really large hands, this may not be for you. Bigger isn't always better! But there are women who can take and want a large, five-fingered lovechild inside them, so if you have a partner who is interested in trying, then lube up and give her a hand!

Psychology of Fisting

Now, if you are not in awe of this eighth wonder of the world, the place from which we all enter it—the vagina—then you are not an ideal candidate to fist one. Fisting takes patience, sweetness, and communication. You must have absolute respect for her body.

♡ Honey, Come Closer

Vaginal fisting requires a delicate balance of two opposites: total surrender and total control. She runs the fist fuck. You must be tuned in to her body's reactions and rhythms, and she has to tell you exactly what she wants. You are her coach, there to support her, encourage her, tell her how good she's doing, tell her how beautiful her pussy is and how amazing it feels wrapped around your hand. That's why we say you must have total pussy appreciation to be a fister of one—your job requires it.

The level of trust between you and your partner is another determiner of a potential fisting session. Penetration *of any kind* is linked to vulnerability, because it takes trust to allow another person to enter one's body. Allowing a partner to reach inside of one's body with their whole hand takes penetration to another level. Be prepared. A lot of emotions could surface during a fisting session, so if you have not established trust with your partner, you are probably not ready to venture into the world of hand love with her.

Willingness and Desire

She must be completely into the experience of being fisted, just as you should be completely into fisting her. *This is absolutely not an activity for someone who is unsure about it.* Remember all that talk in the anatomy chapter about the vaginal and pelvic muscles? If she's unsure or nervous about trying, then her vaginal muscles will likely be tense, making it difficult, if not impossible, for you to get your hand in. That equals pain and discomfort, and most likely an unwillingness to ever try it again.

> *It has to be mutually desired, or it can be frightening. I feel that exclusively fisting a woman without stimulation is not as enjoyable. Slow and easy wins the race.*
> —Beta, 22, Michigan

Really talking it out beforehand will make the experience richer, and troubleshoot potential problems, while alleviating any fears. You can show her this chapter or other information on vaginal fisting to start a dialogue, and see what happens. If she decides she is ready and really wants to go for it and you are the next dedicated candidate for the handball championship, then let the games begin.

The Vaginal-Fisting How-to

Preparation

There are some important preparations to make for a positive hand-love experience. The following list should make you Johnny-on-the-spot.

1. *Talk about what you each want.* Make sure you are both on the same page with what you want from the fisting and how you are going to approach it. Having a conversation prior to getting into it is imperative. Communication throughout the experience is an *essential* element of hand love. Clarity and follow-through will help establish trust, making the experience much richer.

2. *Clip and file your fingernails!* Your fingernails and her vaginal walls are not complementary. Keep that in mind with any finger penetration. Even if you have little nails, they can make minuscule cuts in the vaginal walls. Coupled with lube or her juices, this can make for a stinging vagina and will cut your session short. So clip the nails and file down the edges, since they tend to be even sharper right after they've been clipped. You don't want something silly like fingernails to get in the way of your expression of hand love.

3. *No jewelry.* Obviously, take off all rings and bracelets you might be wearing.

4. *Latex gloves.* Using latex gloves alleviates problems with nails and protects you both from any kind of infection. (If you choose not to use them, make sure you wash your hands thoroughly with antibacterial soap and scrub under your nails before your session. The vagina is highly susceptible to any bacteria that may be hanging out under your fingernails or on your hands.) Some women have allergies either to latex or to the talcum powder that comes sprinkled inside many gloves. The powder can get on the outside and really irritate her vagina. The best way to go is to use nonpowdered gloves or rinse your gloved hands to get any powder off before you start. Do not towel-dry them—towels carry many particles and bacteria that you could introduce to her vagina. During the fisting, if there is any sign of a problem like a rash or swelling, you should stop immediately. It is probably an allergic reaction, and she should rinse off her vulva as best she can to get rid of any residue. If the problem is the latex, gloves made of polyurethane are available. Polyurethane isn't elastic like latex, so these gloves won't fit

as snugly, but they are the next best thing for anyone with latex allergies. Another advantage to gloves is that their slick texture helps your hand glide more smoothly into her vagina. Some women, though, like more friction and gloves can actually impede their pleasure, but save that for advanced hand love. In the beginning, caution is best. Not to mention that latex is sexy for many people. Entertain a latex fetish!

5. *Lubricant.* You will need a big bottle of water-based lubricant—essential! Find out during other activities which lubes she likes that won't cause any funky reactions or discomfort; it's not a good idea to try out a new one during a fisting session. Pump bottles are best, as they are easiest to handle when you're a bit tied up. It is also useful to keep a cup of water close by to rejuvenate your lube when it's drying out—add a drop or two with your fingers, and it will make the lube saucy again.

6. *Towels.* Have a few on hand for the session. You'll want one large one to put under her and one or two more for wiping your hands and her body, unless of course you like getting lube and pussy juice all over everything.

7. *Mirror.* A little stand-up mirror is an excellent accessory to have for your hand-love partner so she can see exactly what you're doing. Prop it up at a good angle so she can see what you are seeing as it is happening. The visual stimulation of watching you enter her may be another element of her turn-on.

8. *Toys.* Make sure that any toys you are going to want are well within reach. You may want some dildos as you prepare her vagina and help it to open up. She may want a vibrator either while you are entering her or once you are inside. Any toys she likes that may add to the pleasure of the experience can be incorporated.

9. *Time.* Fisting is a process that takes some time, especially if you are a novice. It's not quickie material. Make sure you set aside at least an hour and a half for a hand-love session so there is no pressure to finish or reason to rush.

10. *Focus.* A hand-love session requires all of these things and, most of all, complete focus. You must be totally present, sober and aware. You must be focused on your partner and feel connected to her not only physically but mentally and emotionally as well. Like any intimate act, fisting will call up emotions, unexpected psychological responses, and issues of trust and vulnerability in both you and your partner. If you are not 100 percent focused and present, you will not be able to deal with the feelings that crop up, troubleshoot problems, or make your partner feel safe. If you are going to try it, you've got to show up for the occasion on every level.

Get Her Turned On

First off, her vagina has to be prepped, open, and wanting to devour your hand. You don't just dive right into a fisting. When she gets aroused, the vagina elongates and balloons out in the inner third, making it much more able to accommodate a hand. But she has to work up to this state. The vagina is not automatically ready for a fist. You have to seduce it first.

Try starting with a bath, to get her blood flowing and her body warm, cleansed, and relaxed—water is a romantic and appropriate element to incorporate. Don't use any bubbles or smelly things that could get in her vagina and cause irritation later. Basic Epsom salts are probably the furthest you want to go with the bath accoutrements because they are mild and help the body relax.

Start with lots of kissing, get her all hot and bothered, then stroke or lick her vulva. Some fucking might be good, but if you are going to have intercourse, think about what contraceptive method you are using. It wouldn't be wise to use a diaphragm or a cervical cap, as you wouldn't want one inside her vagina when fisting her—it would likely get dislodged and thus would not be reliable. Condoms or a hormonal method would be best for a hand-love session. It may not be a good idea to introduce any outside fluids (like your semen) at all, especially if she is prone to any vaginal or urinary-tract infections.

We don't want you to deplete your energy, so you can also use a variety of dildos. Start with a smaller one and work up to a larger one before attempting to put your hand in her juicy, turned-on pussy. Whatever it is she tends to like as far as vaginal penetration goes, you are going to push the envelope further than usual. Just don't wear her out before you even get to your hand.

Find a Comfortable Position

When you are ready to move into the fisting, you want to be in a position that will be comfortable for both of you. She may want to be reclined on some pillows to give you good access to her pussy. If she likes to be on all fours for vaginal penetration, that can work too, as long as she is comfortable staying that way for a while. It is possible to change positions in the midst of inserting a hand in her vagina, but it is tricky and should be reserved for the experienced fister. Whatever the position, your hand needs to go in her with your palm facing the front of her pelvis so it is in line with the curve of her vaginal canal. So if she's on her back, your palm will be faceup; if she's on all fours or propped up on pillows stomach down, your palm would be facedown. Take care that your arm or wrist doesn't end up in a position that will give you cricks or spasms. Make sure you have good light so you can see what you are doing.

Hand Insertion

It will be your job to check in with her during your hand-lovin' session, as she may get preoccupied with all of the intense sensations happening in her pelvis. Ask her things like "How does this feel?" "Should I add another finger?" "More lube?" "Is this okay?" Watch her reactions. If she has any facial contortions that tell you something isn't feeling right, find out how you can correct the problem. Ask questions, and be as specific as you can about what she likes and doesn't like. If at any time she wants you to stop or it gets too painful, then STOP!

:♡: **Honey, Come Closer**

In fisting she has got to call the shots. Let her tell you what she wants when she wants it. Start with one finger, add a second, a third, and a fourth, one at a time. It's best for her to ask for each one as she wants it. Keep a clear line of communication. This cannot be stressed enough. Half of fisting is communication. This should absolutely not be a silent sexual endeavor or one done in the dark.

It is the ultimate feeling of being within someone's being. You have to go very slowly, use a lot of lube, one finger and slowly add more, then all five, then gently push and curl and for God's sake, ask questions and communicate!
—Denise, 24, Queens, New York

As you put each new finger in, add more lube. There are women who don't like lube (or like just a little) because it takes away from the friction of the hand and decreases their enjoyment. The rule of hand is to use copious lube unless she tells you different. Most women will want it, and better to use too much than not enough, especially if she's never been fisted before and neither of you can be sure how her body will respond. This is where that pump bottle will come in very handy—you can pump the lube right onto your inserting hand and fingers with your free hand.

Your knuckles are the widest part of your hand, and the most challenging part to insert. Once all four fingers and thumb are in, you want to cup your hand (like you want to hold water in it), curling it inward as much as possible to create as narrow a knuckle space as you can. Go slow. When she's ready, ease your hand into her. Have her take a deep breath and, as she exhales, push in. Use a little more pressure each time you push, slowly working your knuckles through her vaginal sphincter muscle.

You may not get your entire hand inside the first time. With some women, it might not happen at all. That's okay. Don't force it if it gets too uncomfortable and she doesn't want to go any further. You can only go as far as she is comfortably able to go. Just having all of your fingers in her is a pleasurable and connective act.

Remember, you are her coach. Walk her through what you are doing as you do it. "Okay, I'm up to my knuckles now. This part will be the hardest. I want you to take a deep breath, and I'm going to ease in. Tell me if it gets uncomfortable." Sometimes people forget to breathe, and reminders are incredibly helpful. If you can communicate with her in this way, she will feel safe and she will feel confident in you, which will help her relax.

> *The partners who have fisted me knew what they were doing. The communication involved, the connection, is what makes it so amazing. For me, it's an intensely emotional experience that usually makes me cry. I can't share that with just anyone. I don't think it's for everyone. I think a woman really has to be ready for a fisting, and she needs to have a partner who will really listen, go slow, communicate, and appreciate it.*
> —Jasmine, 30, Chapel Hill, North Carolina

There is likely to be some discomfort and maybe a little pain. It's that pleasure-pain nexus that a lot of people get off on. It's a good idea to keep a vibrator nearby—using it on her clitoris while you are working your way in to focus her attention on another area of pleasure may help. Some women will prefer to totally focus on what your hand is doing and won't want their attention diverted. Others will appreciate it. Do whatever works for her. If she does experience some pain and it isn't a "good pain" anymore, or if it becomes too overwhelming, then don't push her beyond where she feels she wants to go.

If she's fine and wants to keep going, then hang in there with constant check-ins. When you are at the point where you just have to push your hand through, have her take deep breaths, and push in as she exhales. Each time she takes in a deep breath it relaxes her vaginal muscles more, and will aid you as you work your hand inside.

Curl and Tuck

If you are able to get your whole hand in, it will naturally make a fist because your open hand won't fit once inside. As your hand curls, you want your thumb tucked underneath your fingers or it will stick out and be uncomfortable for her. If your thumb ends up on the outside, rest your hand a moment to let her take in the sensations and get used to it being inside her. Then, when she is ready, tell her you are going to tuck your thumb under your fingers. This could be uncomfortable for her, so be gentle and keep your movements as minimal as possible.

Once her vagina is filled with your hand, she is going to feel every movement you make, so do not make quick or jerky motions at any time. Keep this in mind and continue to coach her. Tell her what you are doing as you do it. She will feel a lot of sensations but will not necessarily be able to tell exactly what you are doing, so it is helpful for you to explain as you go.

Visiting Hours with the Womb

Congratulations! You are now inside one of the miracles of the world, feeling firsthand its warm energy radiating out and enveloping you.

Once your thumb is tucked, you've taken some adjustment time, and she is feeling fine, ask her what she wants, and experiment. "Should I keep my hand still, or would you like me to rock in and out a bit?" To rock her, gently move your fist back and forth inside her. You may be able to move it only an inch or so, depending on her shape. She may just want to feel you inside her as waves of energy wash over you both. You will feel a totally new connection to her—her heart beating in her vagina, yours beating in your hand, meshed in her pelvis. You may not even be able to tell whose heartbeat is whose. This is a good time to take a moment to connect emotionally with your partner and look into her eyes if you are in a position to do so.

:♡: Honey, Come Closer

Once inside your partner, take some time to quietly tune in to the feelings in your own body, how being there affects you. Look at her engorged with blood, wrapped around your forearm. See how the colors have changed because of the blood flow and her arousal. What do her vaginal walls feel like? Your arm ends where her pussy begins, and you are linked as never before. Take it all in, honey.

If she's fine and seems to be really loving it, then follow your instincts and do what feels right to you. Be careful with her cervix, and remember, the vaginal tissues are sensitive.

> *It is a unique and powerful experience to share with a partner. The first time I was fisted was the first time I ever cried and became emotional in that way during penetration of any kind. I have found that fisting is one of the best ways to learn about your partner and yourself. A great relationship builder!* —Jennie, 26, Brooklyn

Tears do not necessarily mean she is in pain. Do not misconstrue them. She may be overcome by her emotional and physical connection to you, by the feeling of being so deeply penetrated, or by the stretching of her psychological and physical boundaries. As we've discussed before, when she is penetrated physically, she may also be penetrated emotionally. It's powerful stuff, not for the meek.

> ### :♡: **Honey, Come Closer**
>
> Don't be surprised if she sheds some tears during fist-
> ing. It takes a lot of trust on her part to participate in
> such an intimate and intense act. If she does have an
> emotional release, it's all part of the hand-love session.
> Embrace whatever emotions come up in yourself and
> in your partner, and experience them together.

Orgasms from the Inside

During fisting, she may want to use her vibrator or her hand
to stimulate her clitoris. If she has an orgasm while wrapped
around your hand, you will have a whole new perception of orgasm. Her muscles will contract and release in powerful spasms
around your hand. You will be inside her own personal earth-
quake. How luscious! You've felt the sensation around your penis; this will take it to another level. It should give you an
increased awareness of what goes on in her body throughout
her arousal process. Enjoy it, be sensitive to it, really focus and
appreciate every muscle movement and sensation.

There's a chance that her orgasm will make your hand spasm;
if this happens, just be patient and stay with her. *You should
never try to yank your hand out*—her vaginal muscles will be
contracting, and it could be painful for both of you. You don't
want any broken bones, do you? It has been known to happen.
It's not common, but remember that women's vaginal contractions are powerful enough to push out a baby. You will just
have to wait for an opportune moment, and that moment would
not be in the middle of an orgasm. The calmer you are and the
more your hand relaxes, the easier it will be to ride out the waves.

Coming Out

She may get to a point where she can't take another minute
of the full sensations in her pussy and wants you to come out.
You could get a hand cramp, or your hand might just need a

break. Whatever the reason, when it's time to finish, the fisting must end. Use the same rules of thumb for coming out as you did going in. Don't rush it, don't force anything too much, communicate, and coach her to breathe and relax.

When you are about to come out, guide her through it. "Okay, I'm going to pull my hand out now. I want you to take some deep breaths." Have her breathe deeply for a minute or two before beginning to pull. You want to feel all of her vaginal muscles relax. Usually, each breath will relax the muscles a little bit more. When you're both ready, as she exhales, bring your hand back through the opening in one swift but gentle motion. You want to open and cup your hand to make it as narrow as possible, as you did going in. She may feel some discomfort as you pull out, so make the motion brief. It's like pulling a Band-Aid off hairy skin: The quicker you do it, the less time there is to think about it and the less pain the brain will register. Don't yank it, of course! But don't be timid. Just gently pull. Once you get the knuckles through, your whole hand will be pushed out, emerging on the other side, as her vaginal walls relax.

Afterglow

Both your hand and her pussy will probably be pulsating from all the entwinement and intense sensations they just experienced. Allow them both to rest a bit. Your hand may be pruny or stiff and will probably need some stretching out. Her vulva will be pulsating and warm and will probably need a break.

If she didn't have an orgasm while you were inside, now might be the time for one, so her muscles can go into total relaxation. A little mouth love might be a good choice, although the lube might not taste so good. Rinse it off with water. How about a hummer to sing her praises?

A hand-love session is about her sacred space. It's a different experience from other types of sex, so don't expect any tit for tat. You may be surprised at how much pleasure you get out of a sexual experience that doesn't involve your dick. Chances are, you will both be pretty exhausted, and you might just want to hold each other for a while and stay with the connection you feel. Should you and your lover choose to try it, your first hand-love session will be an initiation you will not forget.

☀ What's the Kink?

As we have discussed, many lesbians are sexually creative people who tend to explore their options. Women lovin' women are no strangers to whips and leather. "Leather dykes" come in all shapes and sizes and intentionally present themselves in leather garb to show their appreciation for this sensual world of pleasure. As wonderful as sadomasochism (S/M), or kink, can be, it takes a lot of work. Not everyone supports, participates in, or likes S/M, but many people do. "Different strokes for different folks."

Variations on kink are D/S (dominance and submission) and B & D (bondage and discipline). These arts include playing explicitly with power within an erotic context, enacting fantasies, exploring pain, or engaging in fetishes. These practices express and explore an erotic art that, like toys and fisting, can be misunderstood and given a bad rap.

For reasons of space, this will not be an exhaustive discussion of S/M, to which many books have been devoted. If you are interested in learning more about it, check out some of the references in the resource list found at the end of this book. You can also seek out clubs where S/M is practiced to check out other players. There are S/M and kink communities in many urban areas. Lesbians, gay men, heterosexuals, and other pansexual people make up the S/M community.

The Myth of Kink

People who engage in any type of S/M activities are typically pegged as freaks, perverted, violent, or sexually frustrated, but it's simplistic to judge others' sexuality based on how far it deviates from our own, calling it sick and deviant because it's not what we know.

But have you ever felt the erotic charge of being held down or of holding your lover down while you were having sex? Known the titillation of being blindfolded by a lover? Ever been tied up? Felt the power surge of putting a lover in handcuffs? Ever given a lover a spanking, or been spanked yourself? Ever pinched a lover's nipples? Even some of the tamest people have participated in these acts.

> ### ☼♡☼ Honey, Come Closer
>
> Tell you a secret . . . most people have engaged in some sort of S/M, bondage, or other D/S activity at some point in their sexual lives. These arts play explicitly with power within an erotic context, and they have something for everyone.

I like a little rough fun—spanking, bites, pinches. It makes the soft kisses even sweeter.
— Angela, 31, Syracuse, New York

Hopefully, by thinking about S/M broadly and in the context of power exchange, myths can be broken down. We all play with power within several contexts. It is an intrinsic part of sexuality. For example, who is on top during intercourse? Who initiates sex in the relationship and when? S/M takes the exploration of power a step further and creates a space where people can *safely* engage in power exchange. It allows people to act out their deepest, kinkiest fantasies in a safe and controlled context.

Roles and Terms

In an S/M scene people play roles and take on personas. A "scene" is a session that two or more players create and play out. There are two basic roles: the "top" —the one who guides, inflicts pain, or dominates the scene (a.k.a. the "dominant," "Master," or sadist)—and the "bottom" ("submissive," "slave," or masochist). The bottom submits to the top, has naughty things done to him or her, or has pain inflicted because it brings pleasure. In any scene there is at least one top and one bottom. Sometimes in group scenes more than one top might take on a bottom, or vice versa. Some people are strictly tops, some strictly bottoms, and those who like to play both roles at different times are called "switches."

> *I like being told what to do, how, and where. I like to make my top proud that they are with me. I like being tied up, flogged, smacked, waxed, and verbally taunted with a touch of humiliation. I like getting scantily dressed and showing off my submissiveness and my body in a scene or club.*
> —Janis, 25, San Francisco

Why People Play

There are endless reasons why people engage in S/M play. Some like to play with pleasure and pain and push their body or their partner's body to the outer limits. They do this within a safe context, where they can stop the scene at any time if it gets to be too much. S/M is an outlet for people to release emotions they can't or don't feel free to in other ways. For people who play in public, S/M is a way to let their exhibitionist selves come out before the appreciative gazes of voyeurs. S/M allows people to explore facets of themselves that they might never have the opportunity to otherwise.

Rules

There are always rules for S/M play. The mantra in the community is "Safe, sane, and consensual" —all very important. It is not always possible to tell if a bottom (or top) is being pushed beyond his/her limits, so a "safe word" determined beforehand by the partners gives her or him the power to stop or slow down a scene at any time. When s/he hears it spoken, the top should respond immediately.

"Sane" means that a scene is for everyone's pleasure. It should not abuse the submissive's vulnerability or otherwise cause emotional harm. A submissive should not have to worry that their top will go beyond his/her limits without consent. The top should always be comfortable with what s/he is doing to the bottom. "Sane" also means that when people play, they are sober. It is downright dangerous to engage in S/M activities while inebriated. Any reputable S/M club will have strict policies about the use of drugs or alcohol by people who come to play.

S/M play must always be consensual. All parties must *want* to play and agree on *how* they will play. Sadomasochism should never, ever be forced on an unwilling partner. Then it becomes assault.

A top and bottom should always negotiate a scene before engaging in any play—discuss what they like and don't like, what they would like to explore, and where their boundaries are. Before you attempt a scene, it is important to ask a lot of questions and be thorough and clear about what you want. Sharing this information is crucial so that the scene will be a positive and pleasurable experience for both parties. After negotiation, the bottom will entrust his or her body to the top and the top must trust that the bottom will communicate limits and desires.

S/M is about playing with boundaries. When you explore boundaries, you may step over someone's limits at some point, especially if they aren't sure what those limits are. There are consequences both positive and negative to S/M play. Sometimes people can get pushed too far and have a strong emotional reaction, so it's important to be prepared to deal with that.

Always check in with your partner. If you are topping your partner and you sense something is going on, ask her what she needs and give it to her. Your partner may need a break, some water, to be held or untied, or to end the scene altogether. Respond immediately, and check your ego at the door. Just because someone reacts in a way you didn't expect doesn't mean you did anything wrong. As long as you check in with your partner and respond to her needs then you've done your part.

> ### ⦂♡⦂ Honey, Come Closer
>
> S/M actually requires more trust than most other sexual exchanges. It involves a high level of communication, so it is probably not for someone who can't communicate about sex very well, since *clear communication is a necessity.* It is the only way to have boundaries respected and players feeling safe.

Psychological Aspects of Power

> *I bought a pair of white stilettos, and my boyfriend started licking them and sucking them and it just drove me nuts. It gave me this sense of power, and I turned into a wild woman.*   —Lissette, 24, New York

Power is an intrinsic part of any form of eroticism. Who has power? Who shares it? Who gives it up? Usually it is shared, but not always. One person might take control for a while, and at some point the other could flip the tables by flipping their partner.

The power we have or don't have in our daily lives often plays itself out in one way or another in our sexual and erotic lives. Often it is the CEOs and other people who have lots of power in their career or in their daily lives who want to be dominated in sex play. They make so many decisions in their routine lives that they need an outlet where someone else takes control and they don't have to do anything but be taken. This is one of many examples of how power feeds S/M from other spaces in our lives.

Gender can be a major component of S/M. Because of the power dynamic it represents, many women may not want to bottom for a man but would for another woman. Or they might bottom or top only for specific kinds of men or women. A woman in one of our groups explained that while she might really get off on being thrown up against a wall and fucked by a woman, she probably would never want that from a man. Many men may feel uncomfortable topping women because they themselves do not like the power structure it represents.

Race and ethnicity can have a similar effect on people. Some people of color may not want to submit to Caucasians because of the inherent power dynamics, while others choose to explore that bottom space with various tops. Like everything else, all of this is individual, and outside forces do affect us.

Depending on people's life experience, their buttons about power can be easily pushed with S/M. It's important to be aware of what buttons you and your partners have, so you can avoid pushing them, or so you can discuss them to see if you want to push the envelope a bit and explore those boundaries. Most people, particularly women and people of color, have been abused by someone else's power over them at some point in their lives, whether at home, at school, on the job, or in the larger context of society. It's important to be aware of what you may represent to your partners when it comes to power.

S/M Basics

There are endless possibilities when it comes to sado-masochistic play. We will outline a few of the basics here to get you started, but we recommend you do further research if you find yourself really interested in inaugurating yourself into the vast world of S/M, D/S, leather, or kink.

Role Play

I use masks a lot. Not leather masks—oriental or elegant character masks, like the devil or a dragon or demon or whatever. Then I put myself in that persona as much as possible for her to experience sex with a creature other than human. —Eric, 22, Roanoke, Virginia

Many people like to explore their kinky side through role play. In a scene you can be whoever you want to be. Role-play relationships can be things like teacher/student, photographer/model, mommy/daddy/girl or boy, mistress/servant, doctor/patient, two children exploring their genitals, or teens on their first date.

> *I role-play a lot more these days. In sexual encounters I like to make up stories or take on a voice or theme. I especially love to act like a "little slut" with my partner. Sometimes we pretend we are 15 or 16, in a parent's house, not wanting to get caught having sex. It's fun.*
>
> —Tara, 26, Albuquerque

You can be any age, gender, person, or creature you want. The possibilities are as vast as your imagination; S/M is a way to exercise it. Anything you imagine, you can create. Your fantasies can come to life with the right partner. Whatever goes on in the fantastic annals of your mind can be brought out, shared, and explored. Dress up, get your props, set the scene, and build the tension. It's better than writing a story—it's acting it out and starring in it. Who do you want to be?

Fetishes

A fetish is any thing or act that is a consistent turn-on for a person. Some folks have a shoe or foot fetish, some have a spanking fetish, some have a breast or penis fetish, a peeing fetish, a leather or latex fetish. We may fetishize things in our daily lives like cars, books, or records. When someone entertains a sexual fetish, that object or act can be a source of arousal, and whole scenes can be created and enacted around it. Some people always need some representation of their fetish present in order to come.

Bondage

Bondage is a common way to explore erotic power. Restraining somebody is a way to feel the responsibility and empowerment of having a bottom at your mercy. And many people get a charge out of being restrained. Any bondage act requires a lot of trust and negotiation beforehand of how the power will be used.

> *I love being tied up. There's something that turns me on about being powerless, having my girlfriend be able to do whatever she wants to me.* —Melissa, 24, London

You may have engaged in some bondage in the past. Many people have been held down or held a lover down for the erotic thrill of the dominance and submission involved. Bondage can be that simple, or it can be much more elaborate as part of a scene or role play. It is often coupled with teasing, punishment, or humiliation, depending on what the players are into. Role-play scenes that would provide a good setting for bondage are endless. Teacher/student, master/slave, police officer/arrestee, kidnapper/hostage. Use your imagination and create a story.

> *I like to be handcuffed to the bed and be taken advantage of, but only if I completely trust the person. I enjoy the loss of control and the communication.*
> —Katie, 28, Portland, Oregon

Handcuffs, leather restraints, rope, or special metal contraptions can be used to restrain someone. If you use rope, you must learn how to tie it properly. As sexy as scarves may be, never use them for bondage as they can tighten and cut off circulation in the submissive. Sex-store employees can be very helpful—ask an expert!

Blindfolds

Depriving bottoms of one or more of their senses—most often sight—can intensify any power exchange.

When sight is taken away, the other senses are heightened. A bottom might be blindfolded while the top walks around the room, building the intensity by teasing with the sounds he or she makes. When the blindfolded bottom is touched, the effect will be different because s/he won't know it's coming and there will be an element of surprise and increased anticipation.

Spanking

Many people enjoy a good spanking, whether as giver or receiver. It's very hot to throw your partner over your lap, or be the one bent over for some erotic discipline. The sound of each smack and the feeling of skin slapping skin are what many people like. Being held down and told why you deserve to be spanked can be a psychological turn-on, as can holding someone and punishing them for being naughty. For tops with butt fetishes, having a sexy ass at their beck and call is as hot as it gets!

There are dozens of ways to spank someone: with a belt, a hand, a paddle; while kissing or making love; bent over a table, strapped to a bed, against a wall; bare-assed pants around the ankles, or with a flipped-up dress revealing white cotton panties.

However you do it, there are a few important rules of hand to provide a good spanking.

- Start light and build up the intensity of your smacks. This is especially important if the bottom is new to spankings, as it takes time to build tolerance. And if you are a first-time spanker, you will have to build up hand tolerance as well.
- *Never* hit her tailbone or anywhere along the spine—keep to the fleshy cheeks.
- Turn the other cheek. Spank both of them. Don't leave one starved for affection.
- If you give her a slew of hits in a row in the same place,

that will be a stinger, so make sure you follow it with some soft little taps or caressing. It's good to mix it up between more intense slaps and your soothing hand rubbing her bum as the slaps set in.

- While it's good to move around the buttocks, you may want to focus some extra attention on the "sweet spot" where the butt cheeks meet the thighs. A higher concentration of nerve endings here makes it oh so sensitive.
- Pay close attention. As with any D/S play, be sensitive to and respect the submissive's limits.

When you negotiate a spanking beforehand, be clear about limits and boundaries. Spankings can leave bruises. For some submissives, having marks left on their bodies is part of the turn-on. They are a "badge of honor" to remember their scene with. But many people don't like to be marked at all, and if that's the case, use caution and go easy. If the skin begins to get really red and welts up, chances are she'll end up with some marks.

> ### ⟨♡⟩ Honey, Come Closer
>
> The best way to be a good spanker is to get spanked. The way to be a good top is to bottom, so you know firsthand what it feels like when you do naughty things to your bottom. Tell her you have been a bad boy and roll over!

Spankings are often part of role play, especially where one person plays younger. Again, this has to be negotiated, because most people have psychological limits as to how young a character they can play. If you are dealing with someone who was sexually or physically abused as a child, a spanking could trigger something in them they may not be prepared to deal with. Be cautious about the roles you choose. Make it fun and respect limits. For many people spanking is as far as their S/M exploration will ever go. Spanking can be incorporated into sex or stand on its own as an erotic act. Sometimes a bottom can even reach orgasm when turned over a lap because of friction on the genitals. S/he may need to be punished for that!

Expanding Erotic Knowledge

Through S/M with a willing and enthusiastic partner, you can explore sides of yourself that you normally keep locked up. Try reversing roles. If you think you are a dominant, do a scene where you are submissive. See how that feels. You might be surprised. Once people begin, they usually find they are into things they never thought they would be. Sometimes fetishes reveal themselves in totally unexpected ways. Exploring other sides of your nature is an opportunity to expand your awareness as a lover and as a human being.

Tying It Up

Heavy S/M play is not for most folks, whether gay or heterosexual. It's a different kind of eroticism from "vanilla sex" (sex without any S/M or kinky activities). Some people may dabble in S/M a bit and decide it's not for them, or just do it once in a while, while others may invest in a whole wardrobe of costumes, start a whip collection, and make a lifestyle out of it. Many people may simply explore their own personal fetish and keep it simple. S/M may or may not include "straight" sex.

You may never explore S/M yourself, but hopefully you can understand why some people are attracted to it. It's a way of pushing boundaries in a safe context. Some people go sky-diving; others like to be bound and tortured. As long as it brings them pleasure, it's consensual, and safety precautions are observed, it can be a mutually positive and satisfying experience. If you are seriously interested in exploring S/M, check out some of the books on the market (there are a few on our resource list) that discuss it at more length.

Roadblocks

☀ Detours

Roadblocks and conflicts can be resolved in a way that takes your love life to a higher level, or they can destroy a relationship. The roadblocks in this final section are discussed in a general way. They can affect any relationship, regardless of gender. There is not a uniquely "lesbian" way to handle these situations. We wanted to include this as a basic primer to acknowledge that other issues will affect your sexual relationship and create barriers. These are some guidelines for everybody and this is not an extensive list as there are many more issues that could come up. Again, we come back to the mantras of communication and trust. Review our communication tips when dealing with the following issues. There are bridges you may have to cross. If the relationship is important to you, it is worth working through the roadblocks with your partner. You might get stymied in traffic for a while, but if you are patient and can get through it, the open road awaits you.

Our Bodies, Not Ourselves

It's a beautiful day, and you're driving your new car with the top down. You just got a raise at work, and you're on your way to your first vacation in five years, a week on a Caribbean beach. With the wind flying through your hair you slow down to pass the car in front of you and notice the bumper sticker, which reads NO SMALL DICKS.

Like most men, you're a little insecure about the size of yours. Suddenly, in your mind, you've become a sexual reject who will never be able to satisfy a woman. Even if your dick is average, who wants to be average? Your heart feels like it's been skewered, your self-esteem vanishes, and all the joy goes out of your trip before you even make it to the airport.

Never happened, did it? And it probably won't, because there is no male equivalent of the experience of driving down the street and seeing a NO FAT CHICKS bumper sticker on a car. Few would dream of making nasty public remarks to an overweight man. What would that feel like? Hard to wrap your brain around that one, but you can be assured, it would feel pretty humiliating, especially if it played on an insecurity you already have.

Talking About Her Body

Your partner may place a different interpretation on many things you say, especially when it relates to her body or any insecurities she has about it, so be extremely careful about the words you use. When a woman asks if she looks fat, she wants an honest *and* flattering answer. Don't ever say, "I like you just the way you are." Regardless of how your partner actually looks or how you feel, your "compliment" will be interpreted as if you're lowering your standards to accommodate her imperfect body.

There are other faux-pas responses, but the worst has to be: "Well, honey, there's just more of you to love."

If it seems like a no-win situation, you can turn it around by saying, "You are beautiful," then proceed to gently touch all the areas she is self-conscious about. The more compliments you give her, the more attractive, confident, and sexually desirable she will feel and *be*.

> *I have a friend whose father always told her she had a fat ass. You can be sure it's the bane of her existence. It's a double shame when the most powerful men in our lives shame us.*   —Mary, 29, Boston

"Do I look fat?" is a question that can not only destroy the moment—it can kill a relationship. Yet there are few women who have not uttered this phrase at least once in their lives, some every season, and others at least once a day. Our sexual self-esteem can be destroyed by a negative body image. As our society has become more body conscious, both men and women have become more insecure in the bedroom.

> *When I was younger, I wasn't so comfortable getting naked under the glare of lights with someone. Much preferred the lights out, or under-the-covers kind of thing. I'm over that now, though (maybe it comes with age?).*
> —Morgaine, 30, Long Beach, California

Icon Today, Gone Tomorrow

Imagine:

> It is 1950, the year Marilyn Monroe is the archetype of sensuality that Madonna and supermodels have become in the '90s. Like most guys, you masturbate pretty regularly and you like a little visual stimulation for your jack-off fantasy. In fact, in your life to date, you've worked your way through a few thousand issues of Playboy and Swank. Then, sadly, you come down with a terminal disease caused by excessive masturbation. Being a visionary, you decide to have yourself cryogenically stabilized—frozen—until science discovers a cure. And it does!
>
> Today, at the turn of the millennium, you are thawed and sent out into the world, where you stop at a newsstand, pick up a dazzling array of porn, and head to your bed for your first jack-off session in half a century. You open the magazines and the hard-on you've already worked up fizzles at the sight of bizarre, hyperslender, otherworldly alien forms, clearly female, but much different from what you remember. They look like nothing you've ever encountered between the sheets, and you wonder where they came from and what sex with them might be like.

The icons men are served up today are starved, airbrushed, and silicone injected. Imagine being a woman about to take her clothes off for the first time in front of a man she hopes will love her but who she knows has been raised on the "ideal"—retouched, breast-implanted *Penthouse* babes that no biological woman can live up to. As a culture, we are addicted to an unrealistic (not to mention unhealthy) idea of beauty, instead of embracing the diverse, real bodies the vast majority of us live in.

What Goes Around Comes Around

You guys should be able to empathize, because the tables are starting to turn. With Calvin Klein underwear ads and the nation-wide obsession with love handles (or the lack thereof), more and more pressure is being put on you to be not just rich and powerful but trim and beautiful as well. You are made to feel shame if you don't have an abdominal six pack. And even scarier, with the increased popularity of penis-enlargement operations, the day might come when you just won't measure up unless you go under the knife.

Are men insensitive louts who treat women they don't know or women whose bodies don't fit their juvenile fantasy image with less than the respect and kindness they'd give a dog? Yup, a lot of the time. Do they have a lock on loutishness? Imagine the tables turned . . .

> At 13, my best friend and I found a description of the erection process in a book in her folks' library, and we read it over. Neither of us had a brother, and we'd never seen a dick or a picture of one. We were fascinated by the concept of something we'd never seen. One day we got caught in homeroom by some of the boys we considered cute, talking about penises. The boys treated us with a whole different kind of interest and somehow, maybe from some past-life memory, we rose to the occasion by slyly intimating that we'd been keeping a list.

This phantom list, which we hinted at by not very subtly eyeballing each boy's crotch, was a two-woman survey of seventh-grade cock size and became known as "The List." It bought us a level of coolness we'd never experienced before. The cutest boy in class put his hand on my lap during study hall. I got kissed at the water fountain. My best friend got offers that made my little feel-up and peck pale by comparison. We were the size queens of Roosevelt Junior High, and we reveled in it!

Acceptance

He was turned on by my less-than-perfect body. He loved my ass and hips and less-than-flat belly. That was very sexy, to be wanted that way.   —Kim, 22, Brooklyn

You can give your lover the sweetest gift of all, the gift of self-love and acceptance, through your validation. You can convey it in obvious ways, of course, by not teasing her or even subtly lifting an eyebrow when she orders dessert. Many men chip away at their partner's self-image with negative comments about her body and behavior. Support her healthy appetite rather than encouraging poor eating habits. Try to understand instead of judging.

In the best of all worlds, it might be nice to share appreciation of a gorgeous woman walking down the street with the one you love. But few women feel safe enough or loved enough to react supportively or with amusement when you say, "Jeezus, look at that ass!" about some leggy twenty-year-old in cheek-revealing short-shorts. So be sensitive about gawking, and don't push her buttons.

There is also a lot of unhealthy and negative vulva imagery out there that may play into her feelings about her own genitalia. Women don't see other female genitals very often. The one place a sexually curious or adventurous woman might see a lot of imagery is in stroke books, where the vulva is airbrushed to a homogeneous pinkish hue, denuded of excess body hair, with unopposing, symmetrical lips. Some women have actually had their lips reshaped and shortened, convinced by doctors and nasty partners that theirs were abnormal to begin with. Even the language many women use reflects how uncomfortable they are with their own genitals, commonly referring to them as "down there."

Bottom line: Make her feel positive about her vulva's appearance, a concept you penis-proud guys should be able to embrace. Many women have never had anyone spend time looking at their vulva, describing in detail what makes it so beautiful. Most have been told that it's smelly, mysterious, or gross. Revisit genital show 'n' tell, and do your part to validate the beauty of her genitals.

Real Breasts

Women feel the same pressure about breast size that men feel about penis size. Both are empty cultural measures of our worth as sexual creatures. Why else would breast implants be such a booming industry? While many men might love a busty woman, most naturally well-endowed females are self-conscious about the size of their breasts. They probably developed early on and were teased relentlessly for having budded early. For this reason, it isn't a good idea to say, "Wow, you are stacked. I never realized your tits were so big." Women with small breasts probably got teased too. There isn't a whole lot of validation for smaller breasts, yet many men and women prefer small perky breasts to large ones. Don't call them "small," just call them "beautiful."

What this all comes down to is quite simple: respect. If you respect your partner and her feelings, you can avoid a lot of unnecessary hurt and discomfort. The best sex happens when you and your partner feel totally comfortable and at ease in your bodies. With that, you can concentrate on what those bodies are doing to each other, instead of feeling judged and self-conscious, which takes energy away from the sexual act. You'd be surprised how open, experimental, horny, and sexy your lover becomes when she feels safe, appreciated, and accepted.

Sexually Transmitted Infections (STIs)

It can happen to any of us. If you are bumping genitals and sharing body fluids with anyone, you could get an STI. It doesn't mean you are bad, irresponsible, dirty, or being punished. It's part of life, and it's part of our responsibility for sex.

If you have a sexually transmitted infection, it's essential that you communicate that fact to your partner for her protection. She should do the same. If you hesitate to speak for fear that the issue could cause problems, imagine the anger and resentment you'll encounter if the infection is passed to your unsuspecting lover. The betrayal will break down any trust you have built faster than you can spin your head. There is no excuse for not being clear on issues of health. If you are dishonest, then you *are* an irresponsible and disrespectful lover. Sure, breaking this news is going to have ramifications. It may scare your partner. She may question your moral character, but having a sexual infection has nothing to do with character. It doesn't mean anybody is a "slut" or "dirty" or "irresponsible"—all it takes is *one* sexual encounter with an infected person. Things happen, even when safety precautions are taken.

Likewise, avoid judgment if your partner has an STI. Neither of your sex lives started when you met, so don't expect her to have no past. If you want to remain in a sexual relationship with her, learn about the STI and how to avoid getting infected, then communicate clearly and take safety precautions. And remember, it's not easy for her either.

> *My partner and I both got HPV—genital warts. Kinda put a damper on sex. We sought treatment and information (perpetually, we're always trying to learn more about it). It made me uncomfortable with my vulva/vagina, which was really upsetting, because I had worked really hard to get to know and love it. It did not come naturally.*
> —Kitty, 21, Westchester County, New York

Sexually transmitted infections are not easy to talk about. Again, review the "More Than Lip Service" section for tips on how to approach a conversation about STIs. Your partner's response in such a conversation offers you a good opportunity to learn about her, and her you—the good, the bad, the ugly. If the conversation is plagued with blame, resentment, and anger, serious and sometimes irreparable damage can be done. However, if it is filled with honesty, understanding, and openness, it could be a major step in building trust and creating a lasting relationship.

Birth Control

Another bridge you will cross is birth control. This is a loaded issue and can be a microcosm of an entire relationship. Who takes responsibility for it? Which contraceptive is used? Is it used responsibly? Are the limitations of that method respected by both partners?

One of the best things you can do as a man—one that will go a long way toward making a woman trust you—is to *share* the responsibility for birth control, get involved in the reproductive health of your partner, and try to carry a little extra weight. This means buying the condoms and sharing the cost of the gynecologist, the pills, the diaphragm, the spermicides. It means going with her to her annual gynecological exam if she wants you to. Some good providers will let you sit in on the actual exam so you can learn more too. This is a great way to build intimacy. She shouldn't have to go it alone. Have her teach you how to insert her diaphragm so you can help. It doesn't have to be an interruption of sex—it can be an erotic part of it.

Don't complain about using a condom—she would love it too if the two of you could go all natural, but you need to be responsible. Use a sheath from your first thrust to the last. Don't put one on halfway through the act. Remember, it protects you too. Condoms are the only birth-control method that also protects both partners from STIs. If you aren't using them with your partner(s), every month becomes a lottery filled with anxiety. Remember, the quality of sex suffers when either partner is concerned and worried about an unwanted pregnancy or getting an STI because your mind is somewhere else.

Also, don't pressure her to use a certain birth-control method. For example, don't pressure her to go on the pill. How would you like to fill your body with hormones day after day? Take a genuine interest and discuss the subject with her, helping her weigh the pros and cons of the methods she is considering. Help her choose the method she feels most comfortable with, and then stay involved by helping her use it effectively so both of you can alleviate worries and focus on good lovin'.

Unintended Pregnancy

Unfortunately, no birth-control method is 100 percent effective 100 percent of the time. Even if you use birth control properly, there is still some risk. Unintended pregnancies do happen. This is one area where most lesbians are off the hook, but women who have sex with men may always have an iota of worry in the back of their mind: Will I get pregnant?

> *I don't know if I was ever pregnant, but I did have to take the morning-after pill once, and I felt so alone. My friends supported me, but no one came with me to the clinic. I think counseling would have helped.*
> —Simone, 23, Phoenix

If your lover gets pregnant unexpectedly, do not run away. Take on some of those lesbian processing skills and discuss the situation with her. Understand that something major is going on in her body and that it may be very upsetting for her. Unplanned pregnancy is scary. Help her weigh the options. If she makes a decision, do all you can to support her in it. Even if you disagree, remember that ultimately it is her body and she will have to live with the consequences of the decision. This doesn't mean that your feelings are not important. They absolutely are, and you should discuss them with her. But her body has gone beyond her control, and she's got to get that control back. A woman must be ready and willing to nurture a fetus in utero and to birth and raise a child, regardless of whether the child's father will be there or not. If you really care about her, you'll be with her through the experience and help her get over the obstacles. A heavy experience like this can certainly bring you a lot closer.

Sexual Invasion

Sexual abuse in our culture has reached epidemic proportions. Unfortunately, the common statistics of assault in women—1 in 3 or 1 in 4 over their lifetime—are probably low. The statistics on men are usually 1 in 7 but are probably even more off because men are less likely to report their assaults. Be assured that there are people in your life who have experienced some kind of sexual assault, rape, or incest and that it will have affected their sexuality in some way. At some point, you will probably have a lover who has been assaulted, and that experience may very well play into your sexual relationship.

> *My sexual assault really affects my sexual interactions and my level of trust and comfort.*   —Michelle, 25, New York

An experience of sexual invasion is carried in the cells of the body. It will be there beneath the surface, ready to be triggered at any time. It is usually during the deepest emotional lovemaking that it will surface.

> *Once when I was having sex with my girlfriend, we were both really getting into it and it was so sensuous and I felt really connected to her. All of a sudden, she stopped cold, her body got stiff, she closed up, and she couldn't speak. I stopped what I was doing and asked her what was wrong. She could barely speak, and I was really concerned. I just waited patiently until she could explain. Finally she said, "I'm sorry. You just moved and touched me in the same way I was touched when I was molested as a child." I had unknowingly awakened her past experience, and I felt so horrible. But I just stayed with her and held her and we*

talked until she didn't want to discuss it anymore. We were able to go back to the loving space we had been in, but it was necessary to stop and deal with the emotions it brought up in her. It upset me to see her in so much pain.
—Kelly, 30, Richmond, Virginia

There tend to be three levels of response when someone has been assaulted sexually. First, the person will be overcome with rage that her body has been invaded and her boundaries have been ignored. Second, she will close down and feel humiliated. Last, she'll feel grief, which often brings on uncontrollable sobbing as she mourns her experience and loss. These responses could come out all at once in a sexual encounter, or they could surface over the course of months or years.

If you have a partner who goes through this while you are having sex, do not get scared and run away. Be there for her. Stay open to her, listen to her, and nurture her through it. Give her whatever she needs, and whatever you do, don't disappear. You will be an immense help to her. Her invasion eroded some of her ability to trust, especially if the perpetrator was someone she knew. If you help her work through it, you may help her reestablish trust. If you run away, you could damage her more. Understand that there may be sexual acts she will not want and adjustments may need to be made. If you have a hard time dealing with the situation, be sure to take time later to acknowledge your response. Follow up and talk further with her. You might also want to seek out someone else to talk with. There should be organizations in your area that can be of service, and remember, it takes time to get through the healing process.

Sex Under the Influence

Many people, gay and straight, engage in sex while under the influence of drugs or alcohol for various reasons. A popular one is that lowering their inhibitions helps them make the moves easier. Some folks think drugs like marijuana or alcohol make them hornier and more relaxed for sex. However, most drugs, including alcohol, actually create physical barriers to sex, such as difficulty in getting or keeping an erection, loss of vaginal lubrication, and a general lack of dexterity.

It's up to each individual to decide whether to engage in sex while drunk or high, but at least be honest with yourself about the possible effects. The biggest problems with being under the influence are that people don't always protect themselves, remember the condoms, or use them properly because their coordination is sloppy. It is well documented that many sexual assaults are related to alcohol or drug use. People aren't as good at respecting other people's boundaries when they aren't sober.

> *I was with this guy who was really into having sex but too loaded to perform. I had a hard time convincing him to let it go (to stop and go to sleep). When I've been with guys who were loaded, it has generally not been a real positive or fun experience.*   —Erica, 31, Dallas

Let's just say that drug and alcohol use isn't going to make you a Casanova, and you may risk pushing boundaries that shouldn't be pushed. The best lovers are sober lovers. You aren't going to be fully present when you are on drugs or alcohol—how could you be?

If one of you has a problem with alcohol or drug addiction, it may have a profound effect on your sex life and will require seeking out resources like a counselor or a sober support group.

Sexual Styles

Perhaps one of the biggest roadblocks to sexual intimacy is when partners have different sexual styles. Sometimes you just have different sexual needs. Conflict can come when one person wants to have sex a lot more than the other. Some people's sex drive is simply stronger than others'. This is true for both lesbians and heterosexuals. The first step, as always, is to talk about it. Each party needs to be sensitive to the other's needs. The partner who wants it more can use masturbation to satiate his/her drive, and the other partner needs to make an effort to be in the mood more or up the frequency some. If one partner doesn't want sex very much, it often has to do with some other problem in the relationship. That will need to be explored. But if that's not it and compromises cannot be reached, a more radical solution could involve opening up the sexual relationship to other partners so the one who needs more can get it. But any nontraditional arrangement is far from easy and has to be done right in order to work.

> *If I have different sexual desires than my partner, we do only what we both want, and we don't try anything the other person is not comfortable with.*
> —Judy, 20, Raleigh, North Carolina

Other areas of style conflict can involve issues of experimentation. One partner might want to try new things: anal play, dildos, S/M, threesomes, swinging, etc. The other may not be as open to the exploration their lover seeks. This can leave one partner trapped in a very traditional sex life that doesn't satisfy and another feeling the pressure of sexual expectations s/he cannot meet.

For a relationship like this to work, both partners must be willing to compromise. "Okay, I'll try dildos and some bondage, but I draw the line at threesomes." Whatever the compromise, both parties need to bend (over and get a spanking).

Issues of rough sex and tender sex can also be a conflict. Some people like it rough most of the time, while others always like it soft and tender. You've got to get back into the dance and continually work on finding each other's rhythms.

Playing with styles also brings up personal issues. One man we spoke to shared a story about how his girlfriend liked rough sex. He liked it too, but often she wanted to go too far. She wanted rough play that he wasn't comfortable with. During sex, he would get caught up in the moment, then become scared that he might really hurt her, which he didn't want to do. Things would get very intense and out of control. The fear of hurting her started to make him avoid sex. Sometimes they would go without sex for months, which left his partner very unhappy. They probably weren't really sexually compatible. Sometimes there isn't much you can do but evolve into a platonic relationship.

These personal issues can make anyone shut down sexually. It's important to pull them out and talk about them, exploring all the options to see if you can find a compromise where your sexual styles can meet. These conflicts and roadblocks are opportunities to build communication and trust. They are also barometers for the relationship. Everyone is different, so you have to discover what turns your partner on. This means talking about your wants and needs. Be willing to adapt, change, and grow. When your partner is willing to listen to your point of view, make compromises, and stick around instead of running away, you know you're on the way to creating something special.

Heading
for the
Wild Frontier

☀ The New Man

So after a whole book of lesbians teaching you how to be the best lover of women you can be, where are you? What will you, the new man, the new lover, be? What new skills and attitudes will you bring to the bedroom and the altar of your lover's body?

What the Women Want

The women we interviewed have some strong opinions and specific suggestions for you. We thought you'd want to hear from them. The following are some choice responses from lesbian, bisexual, and heterosexual women to a few of our survey questions. We give you the women's voices, talking to you frankly about what they need, want, and desire in a lover. Listen up and take note. Many of the complaints are common, and the wishes get wished over and over again.

If you could speak to the heterosexual men of the world about having sex with women, what would you want them to know?

Take time, be patient, LISTEN, ask questions, and be honest.

The sun does not rise and set around your penis. Sex is way more than intercourse, and for a woman, the penetration does not provide the most stimulation. Also, take your time and make the whole thing last.

Be attentive. Ask questions. Be willing to learn.

I generally think they need to talk more and assume less. But to be more specific, here are several tips: cut nails, more foreplay, experiment, don't fall asleep after, orgasm isn't always the goal, be gentle on the clit at first. All of this depends on the woman.

Be more in tune with sounds, like when she's turned on. What it feels like when she's excited: listen to her breathing, ask her what she wants.

Read Joy of Lesbian Sex *or talk to a few lesbians. Mostly, talk to your partner: often, directly, honestly, respectfully. And lighten up and be playful!*

Clit, clit, clit. The old "in and out" just isn't enough. Lots of touching and petting. Foreplay is the key.

RELAX.

Women can have more astounding sex than men and can teach men many things if they're open to learning. Treat your woman well and she'll reciprocate.

Not all women are the same. Notice the nuances.

Be sensitive, know what she wants, and don't always be one-track-minded. It'd be perfectly normal one day to just have a conversation during sex, relax, and you'll still be getting your pleasure out of it, and now, so will she! I would want them to know that we are quite complex. I would want them to know that we are not merely receptacles for their pleasure, but that we are capable of incredible levels of sexual intimacy if we are treated with respect and attentiveness.

SLOW DOWN!

All women are different, and how informed a woman is about sex will determine how good of a sex partner she is. If she is good, it doesn't make her a "ho."

It's okay for women to masturbate and use toys. It doesn't make you inferior.

Be yourselves, be confident, be patient, ask questions, and always make her feel beautiful.

Variety in touching is important, creativity is key, and attentiveness to the other's pleasure principle is of utmost importance.

Pay attention, and use all of your anatomy while having sex with a woman.

Try to obtain her interest in you as a human; it will increase her arousal and subsequently increase the quality of sexual interaction.

Just because you can have sex does not mean that you're a sexual superstar. Some guys think that if a woman sleeps with them, that means that she's totally into him. Women are just as capable of having casual sex as guys are. Don't flatter yourself.

Take a little time and listen to your girl's body.

If they pay attention to their partner, they will be given all the information they need to be a good lover for her—both verbally and nonverbally.

Don't head right for the "naughty bits." Caress, kiss, bite necks and ankles or inner arms. All the skin is a sex organ.

It's not a movie. Your friends aren't watching. It doesn't matter what you look like while you're doing it, just that things feel good. Theatrics don't impress us—moaning, groaning, flexing, etc. Talking about what you like (regardless of how embarrassing) and asking us what feels good is great.

Be patient. Especially when you're going down on a woman. Orgasms don't happen in ten seconds for men OR women.

I would want them to know how important communication is, because every woman is different with regard to what feels good to her. But I think a common desire for women is to have their clitoris stimulated a lot. That's the best, and men, don't quit early. That's a big letdown for the woman. Make sure you know she is satisfied before you stop.

Be open to new ideas. It makes sex much more fun! Perhaps after establishing trust, initiate communication with the woman on what feels good to both of you.

Keep an open mind in your sexual experiences. Try it if she suggests it, even if it sounds weird (you may like it).

Be nice to women! Not all of them are the same—just because you got fucked over by one doesn't mean all women fall under the same category. Make sure she is caring, nice, and wants to be your friend before you have sex.

Go slow, tease, look the woman deeply in the eyes.

Tell us what you want, and we might do it.

Approach the clitoris with care—direct, hard pressure doesn't always work.

Ask. Suggest. Show a picture. Bring it up for discussion. Slow down! Appetizer before the main course.

Know yourself, your body, be comfortable with your body and your sexuality. Learn to appreciate the beauty of a woman's body, of the vulva, vagina, everything! Appreciate the differences.

What frustrates you most about heterosexual men in relation to women?

That they have been so scripted to not listen or communicate with their partners!

When men think they know it all, especially about oral sex, and their need to define sex as a penis-in-vagina with him coming.

That they hurt them physically.

Their need to have their ego stroked and to feel like they have power over women. To put women and their bodies down and assume they [men] are so important and attractive.

Their assumptions. Flirting isn't necessarily a come-on. Sometimes just making out is enough for one night. But primarily men need to relax and see what happens like women do.

Egotism, insensitivity, lack of romanticism. It's not just about "wham, bam, thank you ma'am."

They just don't understand women. I would like to see the more emotional side.

Being emotionally absent. Insensitivity to my mood.

The fact that they don't realize how much of what they say is internalized by women. I have a lot of friends whose husbands can say something hurtful about their physical appearance and not realize what they have done. They are unaware that they are potentially setting these women up for eating disorders and poor self-image. They don't usually do it intentionally, but nevertheless, it's just as damaging.

Sexist and racist comments and attitudes.

Hostility, sexist behavior, condescension, inordinate drinking or smoking.

They do not pick up any subtleties, hints, second intentions, innuendoes.

Disrespect. Any man who thinks he's smarter than you and feels the need to show you. Men who like to play head games to make their women feel inferior. You should be with someone who makes you feel good about who you are, not those who try to make you feel grateful that they would agree to date you.

Arrogance, impoliteness, treating women as sex objects. Thinking he can get anything he wants from me.

Possessiveness, too much dependence (there needs to be a balance between independence and dependence), self-righteousness, arrogance.

Noncommunicative! We are supposed to read their minds!?

What turns you off sexually in a man?

Pushing to have sexual interactions when I'm not in the mood; selfishness.

Being so full of himself that he forgets to ask you what you want or feel.

Guys who don't get foreplay are a drag.

I am incredibly turned off by cockiness. I think humility is incredibly sexy. I am turned off by men who say they are going to call and don't. I am turned off by men who put me last, who assume I will just be around when they have time. I am turned off by men who don't make an effort to make meaningful plans with me but just say, "What are you doing this weekend?" I am turned off by men who find my feminism "cute." I am turned off by men who never compliment me. I am very turned off by men who brag about past sexual exploits. I think men who warn me away from them, saying they are "dangerous," are ridiculous. I think men who ask for my number and won't give me theirs are Neanderthals. Men who insult me EVER are completely out of the question.

Poor hygiene.

I do not like timid men who are nervous or afraid—they do not provide enough stimulation or motivate interactivity. I want to feel him but not feel pain or be treated in a rough or unconcerned manner.

When they are interested in only their own satisfaction, or when they think they know everything and won't take instruction about what I like or how I like to be touched. Some men seem to think all women are the same in bed.

Men who think of their penis as a magic wand and don't use other parts or their full body in making love.

Their inability to let go of ego and preconceived ideas about what women want (like a big penis).

Selfishness. Not being adventurous.

When a man lies there and waits for you to play on him. When a man does something to make you feel good but doesn't do it long enough for you to reach orgasm. When a man only has sexual intercourse with you for the purpose of reaching orgasm for himself and is not concerned with whether you had an orgasm. When a man is afraid to explore or take your ideas with an open mind and try them. Too afraid, or whatever the reason may be.

His not being willing to talk about sex and issues related to it (e.g., STIs, contraception).

What turns me off is guys who are in a hurry, who aren't really into it, guys that aren't open-minded, or guys that do the same thing every time.

When I'm being (or trying to be) intimate with him and I can't tell if he even knows someone else is there. Also, being too "macho"; hypermasculinity is a big turnoff.

Going too fast and satisfying themselves only!

There are definitely trends in the women's sexual frustrations, but we know you aren't in this only for yourself; otherwise, why bother reading this book? But the point is worth stressing, because obviously there are a lot of selfish men out there for all these women to be saying such similar things. Keep your behavior in check.

Now, let's have a little discussion about you and your penis.

How's It Hanging, Boys?

This section is dedicated to the one you love: your penis, your Johnson, your little Marlboro Man, your Cyclops and his two nutty buddies, your joystick. Think a lesbian doesn't know dick about your package? Think again.

We hope to help you develop a healthy and relaxed attitude toward that part of your body that has occupied most of your brainwaves for most of your life. In case you haven't pieced it together yet, we're going to put the mighty phallus in its proper place in the pecking order. Brace yourself for the countdown:

➡ **Your Most Important Sex Tools**

1. Your brain.
2. Your mouth.
3. Your hands.
   (Drum roll, please . . .)
4. Your dick—a distant fourth.

Don't you feel better now—more relaxed—knowing that it doesn't all boil down to your dick? Heave a sigh of relief. You have other tools of love.

Performance Pressure

A man always wonders if he measures up. Not only if he's big enough and good enough in the moment, but how he measures up against former lovers.   —Brad, 27, New York

I feel like a loser if I have an orgasm first.
                              —Jake, 31, Baltimore

Being good in bed always meant intercourse, penetration. Not going down or anything else. The pressure has always surrounded that one act.   —Byron, 37, Boulder, Colorado

So what do most men think of as their most important sex tool? Most would say it is their tool, of course! Oh, the irony! What men perceive to be their most important asset is really one of the lesser in the grand scheme of sex. In fact, to be a great lover, the best thing you can do is forget about your penis. Scandalous but true! Give it up, boys. If a penis is what makes you a great lover, then you'll never be able to hold a candle to a lesbian. She can strap on a dildo of any shape or size, go all night, and never have problems getting it up.

> ### ⭑♡⭑ Honey, Come Closer
>
> You can learn a lot about having a dick by strapping one on. By not being so caught up in your dick's pleasure, you can learn how to better use it to please your lover. And a strap-on is a much more obedient listener!

Your penis has probably caused you more anxiety than it's worth since the first day of gym class, when you got into the compare-and-despair syndrome, seeing who was big, feeling how small you were (it was cold in those showers), seeing who had hair and who didn't. As you got older, the pressures of getting it up and not coming too soon began to fill you with anxiety. It's not that easy having a dick.

When the Plumbing Fails

Many penis problems come from putting too much pressure on yourself to perform, thinking your penis is the alpha and omega of your worth as a human being. The world does not revolve around your cock. Believing this should relieve a lot of the pressure. Your culture has taught you to think about your penis in a certain way, and it's hard to stop. It's hard to change. Awareness is a good start.

Most men struggle with some kind of erection difficulty at some point in their lives. The two main problems are premature ejaculation and not being able to get it up. Relaxing will take a lot of weight off of you, so you can get it up and keep it up longer. What follows is some general advice you can try, and check at the end of this book for other helpful resources.

Leaving the Party Early

With patience and practice, premature ejaculation can often be prevented. It's about knowing yourself and communicating with your partner.

> *Lots of dysfunction with the men I've known in all age groups. Very disheartening. They don't want to talk about it, or they want me to pretend it's all fine. They aren't often willing to learn what they can do for premature ejaculation, for instance.* —Margie, 51, Orlando, Florida

The key requirement for controlling when you come is getting in touch with what is called The Point of No Return. You can work on this with a partner and when you masturbate. This is the moment when you've gone over the edge, you're going to come, and there's nothing in the world that can stop the flood, since all the mechanisms have been set in motion. It's like the first domino has been pushed, and now they're all going to fall. It doesn't matter what you do: stop thrusting, pull out, think of your grandmother. You could stop stimulating yourself and lie completely still. The contractions would still continue, and semen would sputter out unwanted.

To gain some control, you need to become intimately acquainted with The Point and learn how to negotiate with it. You have to reduce the stimulation before you get to that point, because once you're there, it's too late. This means, if you're having intercourse you'll have to slow down and breathe and tell your partner to slow down or be still. Once you're back under control, you can start again. Do the same thing when you masturbate to train your body for partner sex: Excite yourself up to the edge of The Point of No Return, then reduce the stimulation or stop it completely until you have things under control.

As you get better at this you can keep stimulation going while you recover, having heightened waves of pleasure during your sexual journey. It is also helpful to contract your PC muscle as you approach The Point, as this will help you control ejaculation. There are also reports that men can increase the quality of their orgasms and even have multiple orgasms (a phenomenon usually associated with women) through conscious PC work.

> ### ❤ Honey, Come Closer
>
> Men who work with the PC muscle can better control ejaculation and overcome premature ejaculation. This can make vaginal intercourse more enjoyable for both partners.

A Good Man Is Hard to Find

You know the old joke that a good man is hard to find, and a hard man is good to find. This problem often comes back to the pressure to perform.

Trouble getting hard can also rear its head at the beginning of a relationship. At this early stage it's too soon to even call it a problem. It's really quite natural. It takes a while to feel comfortable, safe, and relaxed with a new person.

If the situation persists, you should seek the help of a sex therapist or a doctor. An estimated 50 percent of erection difficulties can be traced to health problems, including those related to stress and abuse of alcohol or drugs (prescription or otherwise). If you are having problems getting hard, especially if you're over forty, it would be wise to get a prostate exam.

> ### ❤ Honey, Come Closer
>
> It's ironic that performance anxiety increases the more head-over-heels infatuated you are. So the one you really want to please may be the one who inflames the problem, because you want everything to be perfect for her.

Once I think about it it's over. It's in my head, I can't get it up, and I don't know how to stop thinking about it.

—Bill, 23, New York

My girlfriend was a big help. She didn't make it a big deal and try extra hard to get me up. She said, "Let's just take it slow." That took off the pressure. —Del, 28, Chicago

Quit focusing on your dick! What does this mean, anyway? It means stop thinking about yourself. It's hard to surrender if you're worried about staying hard. It's hard to surrender if you're always trying to perform. Cocksmanship is usually linked to some preconceived notion of performance and not to being in the moment. Lesbians and Zen masters don't worry about their penis size. Be in the moment. Get in the lovemaking zone. Everything else will follow.

☼♡ Honey, Come Closer

Penetration is about what feels good to your partner—the one being penetrated—not what feels good to you. To be a good lover, forget about your dick and tune in to your partner.

Know Thyself

It's important to know yourself intimately. It's not about being able to pass an anatomy quiz. You might be getting a little defensive right now, thinking something like "Hey, I know my own dick. If I know anything, I know my dick. I even have a name for it." The naming part is cool. Too bad more women don't name their pussies.

You may not know your dick quite as well as you think you do. Your relationship with it might be very similar to your relationship with your neighbor—we'll call him Joe (this could get confusing if your dick is also named Joe). You see him every day and you do the same thing, wave hello. Likewise, you, like many men, may be very familiar with your penis, you see it every day, piss the same way, give it the same number of shakes. There's also a good chance that you masturbate the same way and like to get off with a partner the same way most of the time.

> *My dick feels separate from me most of the time. I guess it's*
> *like any other relationship. I need to take time to listen and*
> *try to understand. I take it for granted.*
> —Steve, 24, San Francisco

To be intimate, you have to explore and try new things when pleasuring yourself and when having partner sex. Get to know yourself for the first time, or reconnect with your old friend. This intimacy and openness is important. It will help you to guide your lover in the intimate act of getting off.

Size

Way too much emphasis gets placed on size. The vast majority of men fall within the average range, and that's probably what feels best to most vaginas. It's "average" simply because it's the range of most men. It doesn't mean your penis gets a "C" grade. Some men are overly endowed, and some are smaller than average. Some women are size queens. Some like small penises. On the off chance that this does become an issue, you'll have to find a way to work it out. Your dick doesn't have to get left out, but if she's wanting more, it takes a big man to strap one on that's the size of her liking. It goes without saying that you will wow her with your mind, mouth, and fingers.

Let's rethink the all-too-common compare-and-despair syndrome. Just as women don't get to see other women's vulvas to marvel at their beauty and variety, most heterosexual men don't get to see a lot of other men's erect penises. Some dicks are long and skinny, others short and fat, and others long and thick. Shape can vary quite a bit. Some cocks are pointier than others, and the heads can be quite different. For example, some penises have big mushroom heads and others have helmetlike heads. Also, it is common practice to circumcise male children, but many men are uncircumcised. Some people like the look of a circumcised penis, and many uncircumcised men report a lot more sensitivity because their foreskin protects the head. Many people like to play with the foreskin too.

Each penis is going to have its own unique features. The biggest variance in cock size is at the flaccid stage, when some men are small and others quite big. But in the erect state, the big often don't get any bigger and the little ones bloom. Lots of times the little ones even get bigger than the flaccidly large penises. Hey, life isn't fair. The other guy gets to strut around the locker room, looking all studly, yet he's pretty average.

> *Having a penis can be such a weird thing. It's never the same. A penis is a wild card. You never know which fellow is going to show up: flaccid, perky, large, hungry, indifferent.*
> —Tom, 31, Los Angeles

❤ Honey, Come Closer

Men are often portrayed as sex-crazed animals who think with their dicks. You've even been chastised in this book. Too much dick hubris is not good. Neither is dick shame. It is important for both men and women to have healthy, positive attitudes about sex, their bodies, their genitals, and each other. Be proud of your penis and your sexuality.

Just keep a healthy attitude and don't get too preoccupied with size and penis performance. Focus on being a good lover, pay attention, and practice enhancing all your skills.

☀ Saddle Up

The Quest for Balance

In the bigger picture, whatever happens in real life, in our relationships, and in the world at large affects our sex lives. That's right—all that inequity, unhappiness, and frustration weasels its way into the bedroom and smears our sheets. What men and women need is more balance. That's the crux of the struggles. Who has power, who shares it, who nurtures, who wears the pants. Maybe part of what women want is for men to be a little more like them. That isn't so bad. They want you to get over the ego and arrogance, be more sensitive, and pay some special attention to them. Is that too much to ask?

There are many ways to look at the quest for balance. You don't have to use New Age language or join a men's group. Think of it in terms of evolution—"Be all that you can be." It's like going through boot camp to become more fully human. Ultimately, striving to live within the limits you *choose* will make you the most honest human being and the best sexual partner you can be. Not the limits society puts on you. Not the limits your parents put on you. Your own. Bust out of that old mold you've been squeezing yourself into, and make your own cake.

> *The oldest god was a woman. Everyone worshipped Mother Earth. During the age of the Goddess the feminine principles ruled the world. We lived in peace and harmony with nature and with each other. Then the male god of the patriarchy came with his sword and took over the world. We've been struggling ever since.*
> —Karen, 41, Apache Junction, Arizona

You can look at this as a myth or as facts of cultural anthropology, but the two main characters in this drama, the masculine and the feminine, are widely accepted as major players in our psyches.

Underneath all the sex advice, this is a book about bringing these opposite forces into greater balance and bridging the gaps between men and women a bit. Moving toward this balance is the only way the world will survive and thrive.

> :♡: **Honey, Come Closer**
>
> If you learn anything from this book, learn this: Let go of any rigidity you are hanging on to for dear life, and allow yourself to go to new places sexually and sensually.

The new man has a balance between his masculine and feminine side. He doesn't always have to be right. He doesn't always have to be in control. He doesn't always have to do all the talking. He doesn't always have to be on top.

Even one of the world's greatest athletes has a strong feminine side. Michael Jordan is open, creative, and spontaneous. In interviews, he constantly talks about keeping a balance between forcing the action and letting the game come to him, getting into the flow. Activating and receiving. The new man is all about flow, being able to move fluidly in and out of different roles, being receptive and open, and not getting stuck in one mode.

The masculine quest has been about freedom, self-sufficiency, and control over nature and other people. These are the qualities our culture has valued—the rugged individual who needs no one and who can conquer nature and the world. Women don't want to be conquered; they want to be respected and loved.

> *Sometimes it feels to me that men and women are just different animals and we will never be compatible.*
> —Ted, 27, Boston

Men and women may be different, but this doesn't mean there can't be change and a greater understanding. The new man needs a courageous woman, and he's got to meet her halfway.

Uncharted Territory and the Open Road

I feel caught in the middle and very confused about sex.
The way I learned about it is now considered wrong. I'm
supposed to ask before I do anything? "No" used to mean
"yes." Have I been that evil?   —Kevin, 40, New York

In the arena of sex and relationships there has never been a
more confusing time. We are like newborn babes learning to walk.
We are falling, and we have the bruises to show for it. There is a big
learning curve when it comes to relating to a woman, especially
when the rules for relationships are constantly changing. It does no
good for men to beat themselves up over things they didn't understand; the important thing is to put their new understanding into
action.

> ### ☼ Honey, Come Closer
>
> The wild frontier is scary. It's a mystery and a chal-
> lenge. Few things are more rewarding and challenging
> than exploring unmapped areas of yourself and your
> lover.

Great sex takes a joint effort. It's not magic. Usually, when it
feels like magic, it's because you worked for it. Our newfound freedom has forced us to confront problems and questions that are at
the heart of what it means to be human, and to discover that there
is another world out there. This is good news for men. It's a world
of equality in power and responsibility. A world where everything
and everyone doesn't have to come at a price. A world that doesn't
revolve around your penis. This means the pressures of always having to be in control, of always having to perform, of always having
to be the leader, of always having to make the first move, of always
having to be the breadwinner, of always having to be strong and
silent, will be a thing of the past.

A fulfilling sex life has a couple of key ingredients: communication and openness. Have the courage to let go of the roles you are used to playing. As we've discussed, this is an arena where lesbians often have an advantage because roles are not so rigidly defined. Letting go allows for experimentation, expansion, and evolution in the way sex is experienced. Surrender to the journey.

Ready to Ride

Well, you've made it through the book. You and your penis got a jolt, and you get major credit for hanging in there and listening to a new perspective. You will be a better lover for it. Are you excited? Relieved? Frustrated? Have you had the chance to put these lesbian lessons into practice yet? Remember, it all starts with yourself, your relationship to your penis and body, and your approach to women.

We want you to be the best lover you can be. We don't want all the old, tired complaints women have about men to apply to you anymore. The women want you to slow down and listen to them. They want you to be more attentive to their needs and touch their clitoris more. They want you to communicate and treat them with respect. It's all pretty basic stuff, but too many men don't even get this far. Hopefully, there are enough useful tools here that you can piece it all together and be her dream lover. She's out there, and she's looking for you. We know you won't be one of those guys who gets his rocks off, shoots his wad, and rolls over to go to sleep, leaving her bitter and unsatisfied. Lesbians know better, and so should you.

Relax into the experience of sex and the journey of your body and hers together. Be a great explorer and try on a new hat. The next opportunity you have, try something with your lover that you've never tried before. Try having sex one day without having intercourse. Try a new position. Try a new sex act. Let her penetrate your butt with her pinky finger. Go down on her for an hour or more. Give her a massage, then go to bed kissing and cuddling. Submit to her completely. Let her tie you up. Be the one to show up naked under a trench coat with flowers in hand. Send her a vibrator wrapped in a bow. Spend an afternoon talking to her about your feelings, how you learned sex, and what sex with her does to you. Whatever is striking you, try it!

Saddle up, head out for the wild frontier, and see where a little exploration takes you. The open road is yours to ride. Love her like she wants to be loved and you will go down in her book as the ultimate dream lover. Get all your body parts and all your senses involved. Most of all, have fun!

RESOURCES

Relationships & Communication

The Erotic Mind: Unlocking the Inner Sources of Sexual Passion and Fulfillment. Jack Morin, Ph.D. (HarperPerennial, New York).
An excellent book on how our psychology, emotions, and self-esteem affect our erotic blueprints.

Getting the Love You Want: A Guide for Couples. Harville Hendrix, Ph.D. (Henry Holt, New York).
Guides you through the different stages of a relationship, concluding with a ten-week relationship course. An insightful book for helping you spot patterns of self-sabotage and for understanding how your family has shaped your relationship habits.

Let's Talk: A Guide to Improving Couple Communication (audiotape). Isadora Alman, M.A., M.F.C.C. (3145 Geary Boulevard, #153, San Francisco, CA 94118).

The Fine Art of Erotic Talk: How to Entice, Excite and Enchant Your Lover with Words. Bonnie Gabriel (Bantam, New York).
A comprehensive guide for talking to your lovers in and out of the bedroom, including sensual games you can play to show your appreciation of one another.

Body and Mind

Full Castrophe Living: Using the Wisdom of Your Body and Mind to Face Stress, Pain, and Illness. Jon Kabat-Zinn, Ph.D. (Dell, New York).

Kabat-Zinn outlines a program for dealing with the stresses of modern life. The program includes lessons in meditation, yoga, and relaxation exercises. He communicates complex and esoteric ideas in clear, simple language.

The Book of Massage. Lucinda Lidell, with Sara Thomas, Carola Beresford Cooke, Anthony Porter. (Gaia Books, Simon & Schuster, New York).

A good introduction to massage basics.

Erotic Massage: The Tantric Touch of Love
The Art of Erotic Massage: Vols. 1 and 2 (videos). Kenneth Ray Stubbs, Ph.D. (Jeremy P. Tarcher/Peguin Putnam, New York).

A sensuous book with a primary focus on genital massage for both pleasure and healing.

Female Sexuality

A New View of A Woman's Body. The Federation of Feminist Women's Health Centers (Feminist Press, West Hollywood, California).

A groundbreaking look at women's sexual and reproductive organs and sexuality, complete with detailed illustrations by Susan Gage. Highly recommended, but can be a difficult book to find. Try feminist or gay bookstores.

The New Our Bodies Ourselves. The Boston Women's Health Book Collective (Touchstone, Simon & Schuster, New York).

It's the classic on women's health, all the way around.

Sex for One: The Joy of Selfloving. Selfloving (video). *Celebrating Orgasm* (video). *Viva la Vulva* (video). Betty Dodson (Order direct by writing: Box 1933 Murray Hill Station, New York, NY 10156; (800) 363-7517; www.bettydodson.com).

Dodson is the Godmother of Masturbation and has probably helped more women find orgasmic happiness than any other single human being. Her classic book and her many videos are full of real, accessible, sex-positive information about women's bodies and pleasure. Check out her website for more details and information.

Femalia. Joanie Blank (Down There Press, San Francisco).

A book of beautiful, tasteful up-close photographs of women's genitals. Even if you've seen many, it's amazing to look at the variety in these vulvas, all in one neat little book.

How to Female Ejaculate (video). Fanny Fatale (Fatale Video/Blush Entertainment, 526 Castro Street, San Francisco, CA 94114; (415) 861-4723).

A video featuring Fanny Fatale, Carol Queen, and others with an educational rap about the G-spot and ejaculation, followed by demonstrations of female ejaculation.

Zen Pussy: A Meditation on Eleven Vulvas (video). *Fire in the Valley: An Intimate Guide to Female Genital Massage* (video). Annie Sprinkle and Joseph Kramer (EroSpirit Research Institute, P.O. Box 3893, Oakland, CA 94609; (510) 428-9063).

Zen Pussy is a unique meditative video with up-close shots of vulvas using the language of breathing in a true pussy meditation.

A vulva-positive video, *Fire in the Valley* gives thorough instruction and demonstration of female genital massage, discusses the benefits and encourages partners to explore the fire's power.

The Clitoral Truth (in press). Rebecca Chalker (7 Stories Press, (800) 596-7437; www.sevenstories.com).

Gives women complete, accurate, and explicitly detailed information about their bodies and sexual response, and provides a framework to enhance sexual experiences.

Male Sexuality

The New Male Sexuality: The Truth About Men, Sex, and Pleasure. Bernie Zilbergeld, Ph.D. (Bantam, New York).

A guide book for helping men through the sexual process, from communication to performance. A good section on common male dysfunctions and how to deal with them.

Sexual Solutions: A Guide for Men and the Women Who Love Them. Michael Castleman (Simon & Schuster, New York).

A practical guide for solving common male sexual problems, with especially helpful information on premature ejaculation and impotence.

The Multi-Orgasmic Man: How Any Man Can Experience Multiple Orgasms and Dramatically Enhance His Sexual Relationship. Mantak Chia and Douglas Abrams Arava (HarperSanFrancisco).

This book contains great exercises to strengthen the sex muscles, control ejaculation, and work consciously with sexual energy, helping men take sex to a higher level.

SEX: A Man's Guide. Stefan Bechtel and Laurence Roy Stains (Berkley, New York).

With a conversational style, designed in user-friendly sections, this book is written for a guy's guy. Packed with information on the many important aspects of a man's sex life.

Circumcision Exposed: Rethinking a Medical and Cultural Tradition. Billy Ray Boyd (The Crossing Press, Freedom, Calif.).

Boyd challenges and questions the cultural acceptance and medical value of male circumcision in a passionate and eye-opening analysis.

The Man's Health Book. Michael Oppenheim, M.D. (Prentice Hall, Princeton, N.J.).

A straightforward reference book addressing important health issues in health care for men, ranging from nutrition and skin care to aging and cancer.

Understanding Male Sexuality. (member.aol.com/Sebringsil/sex.htm).

This text-heavy website is a bit dense but has some good information on everything from arousal, orgasm, and erection problems to sexual preference and relationships.

The Joy of Solo Sex. More Joy . . . An Advanced Guide to Solo Sex. Dr. Harold Litten (Factor Press, P.O. Box 8888, Mobile, AL 36689).
The male equivalent to Dodson, these books offer a healthy look at the pleasures of flying solo.

Oral Sex

The Clitoral Kiss: A Fun Guide to Oral Sex, Oral Massage, and Other Oral Delights. Kenneth Ray Stubbs, Ph.D., with Chyrelle D. Chasen (Secret Garden, P.O. Box 67-KCA, Larkspur, CA 94977-0067).
A lushly illustrated book with dozens of clitoris-pleasing kisses and licks.

Nina Hartley's Guide to Cunnilingus (video). *Advanced Guide to Oral Sex* (video). Nina Hartley (Order from www.adameve.com; or (800) 274-0333).
The first title is a great sex positive video that teaches you the basics: from anatomy and G-spot location to specific techniques for going down. The video also includes a sweet section on genital massage.
The second is similar, but includes information for pleasuring both sexes.

Anal Pleasure

Anal Pleasure and Health. Jack Morin, Ph.D. (Down There Press, San Francisco).
The most comprehensive look at the anus and how to care for it and show it a good time. A classic.

Bend Over Boyfriend (video). *Bend Over Boyfriend II* (video). Featuring Carol Queen.
(Available through Good Vibrations and Toys in Babeland).
Both are educational video how-to's exploring the often taboo

subject of men being penetrated anally by their female partners with actual footage of couples engaged in anal play.

The second has less talk and more action.

Guide to Anal Sex (video). Nina Hartley (www.adameve.com).

This video offers a basic and positive approach to anal sex, stressing techniques for preparing to penetrate and helping your partner relax.

The Ultimate Guide to Anal Sex for Women. Tristan Taormino (Cleis Press, San Francisco).

An excellent book geared especially for women seeking information on anal pleasure.

General Interest Sex Books

The New Good Vibrations Guide to Sex. Cathy Winks and Anne Semans (Cleis Press, San Francisco).

A sex almanac that should be on everyone's bookshelf. Written by two sexperts, it is chock-full of solid information about sex.

All About Birth Control: The Complete Guide. Planned Parenthood Federation of America (Three Rivers Press/Crown).

The lowdown on all types of contraception from rubbers to pills.

The Art of Sexual Ecstasy: The Path of Sacred Sexuality for Western Lovers. Margo Anand (Tarcher, New York).

Anand helps the reader explore the spiritual side of sex by shifting the mind-set of sex to an ongoing process and practice.

The Tao of Love and Sex: The Ancient Chinese Way to Ecstasy. Jolan Chang (Penguin, New York).

A great book for exploring ancient ways of pleasure, with especially good sections on penetration techniques and breathing.

The Great Sex Weekend. Pepper Schwartz, Ph.D., and Janet Lever, Ph.D. (Putnam, New York).

A guide for busy professionals who have a hard time getting motivated.

The Guide to Getting It On. Paul Joannides (Goofy Foot Press, USA).
A straightforward, conversational, and humorous book loaded with practical how-to tips.

Turn Ons: Pleasing Yourself While You Please Your Lover. Lonnie Barbach, Ph.D. (Plume, New York).
Filled with ideas for keeping your sex life exciting, this book is especially good at getting all your senses involved in your love-making.

Expanding Horizons

Good Vibrations: The Complete Guide to Vibrators. Joani Blank (Down There Press, San Francisco).

Carol Queen's Great Vibrations Video. (Available through Good Vibrations).
This hands-on video features Carol Queen discussing the many facets of vibrators, and how to choose 'em and use 'em. Excellent information and some hot demonstration.

The Strap-on Book. A. H. Dion (Greenery Press, 3739 Balboa Avenue, #195, San Francisco, CA 94121; (888) 944-4434; www.bigrock.com/~greenery).

The Topping Book, or Getting Good at Being Bad. The Bottoming Book, or How to Get Terrible Things Done to You by Wonderful People. Dossie Easton and Catherine A. Liszt (Greenery Press, *see above*).
The Topping Book is a great introduction for anyone interested in learning how to be a responsible dominant and have fun doing it. A companion piece to the first book, *The Bottoming Book* is for those who want to learn the joys of submissiveness.

S/M: Sensual Magic. Pat Califia (Masquerade Books, Alyson Publications, New York).

Any book by Pat Califia will provide solid information, and this book is a great introduction to the sensuous world of S/M.

Exhibitionism for the Shy: Show Off, Dress Up and Talk Hot. Carol Queen (Down There Press, San Francisco).

Chock-full of excellent information on opening up your erotic world, getting in touch with your inner exhibitionist, and having fun doing it!

SM 101: A Realistic Introduction. Jay Wiseman (Greenery Press, 3739 Balboa Ave., #195, San Francisco, CA 94121; (888) 944-4434; www.bigrock.com/~greenery).

A Hand in the Bush: The Fine Art of Vaginal Fisting. Deborah Addington (Greenery Press, *see above*).

A thorough, informative, and personal read on all the ins and outs of vaginal fisting. A must-read if you plan to explore this art.

Kink Aware Professionals. (www.bannon.com/~race/kap/).

A resource for seeking out kink-positive, nonjudgmental professionals, therapists and information.

Shopping: Toys and Tools

Adam and Eve (mail-order catalogue)
P.O. Box 800, Carrboro, NC 27510
(800) 765-2326
www.adameve.com

A Woman's Touch
600 Williamson Street, Madison, WI 53703
(888) 621-8880
www.a-womans-touch.com

Come As You Are (retail store and catalogue)
701 Queen Street West
Toronto, Ontario, Canada M6J 1E6 (416) 504-7934

Condomania (retail store and catalogue)
7306 Melrose Ave., Los Angeles, CA
(213) 933-7865

351 Bleeker Street, New York, NY
(212) 691-9442
www.condomania,com

Eve's Garden (retail store and catalogue)
119 West 57th Street, Suite 420
New York, NY 10019-2383
(212) 757-8651; (800) 848-3837

Forbidden Fruit (retail store)
512 Neches, Austin, TX 78701
(512) 487-8358

Good Vibrations (retail store and catalogue)
1220 Valencia Street, San Francisco, CA 94110
(415) 974-8980

2504 San Pablo Ave., Berkeley, CA 94702
(510) 841-8987

Mail order: 938 Howard Street #101, San Francisco, CA 94103
(415) 974-8990; (800) 289-8423
www.goodvibes.com
goodvibe@well.com

Grand Opening!
318 Harvard Street, Suite 32
The Arcade Building
Brookline, MA 02446
(617) 731-2626; (877) 731-2626
www.grandopening.com

It's My Pleasure
4258 SE Hawthorne Boulevard
Portland, OR 97215
(503) 236-0505

Toys in Babeland (retail store and catalog)
(800) 658-9119
711 E. Pike Street, Seattle, WA 98122
(206) 328-2914

94 Rivington Street, New York, NY 10002
(212) 375-1701
www.babeland.com

Erotica and Porn

Good Vibrations Guide to Adult Videos. Cathy Winks (Down There Press, San Francisco).

Libido: The Journal of Sex and Sensibility (P.O. Box 146721, Chicago, IL 60614; (800) 495-1988; www.libidomag.com)

Candida Royalle's *Femme Productions* ((800) 456-LOVE [5683]; www.royalle.com).
   Available through Adam and Eve Productions, *see above*.

Sexual Health Information: Hot Lines, Help Lines, Support Organizations

Safer Sex Page (www.safersex.org)
   Answers your safer-sex questions with information on everything from Reality condoms to a directory of lubes.

Coalition for Positive Sexuality (www.positive.org)
   This site deals with basic sexuality issues and is aimed at young people. Good information without being too text-heavy.

Healthy Sexuality (www.healthgate.com/healthy/sexuality)
   A site devoted to understanding sexual health, with articles on such topics as sexual headaches to celibacy.

Sexual Health Infocenter (www.sexhealth.org/infocenter)
   A great site for general sex information, hands-on techniques,

and ordering toys and videos. Includes a sex tip of the week, a monthly quiz, and surveys.

Sexual Health Network (www.sexualhealth.com)
    A site that addresses the needs of those coping with injuries and disabilities. Also has tips on achieving orgasm and getting in the mood. A great site for anyone.

Society of Human Sexuality (www.sexuality.org)
    An online collection of well-written articles from the people at the Society of Human Sexuality at the University of Washington.

STD Homepage (www.grin.net/~sycamore/std/index.html)

National STD Hotline (800) 227-8922

National AIDS Hotline (800) 342-AIDS [2437]

Planned Parenthood (800) 230-PLAN [7526]

San Francisco Sex Information
    P.O. Box 881254
    San Francisco, CA 94188-1254
    (415) 989-7374
    www.sfsi.org

The Sex Institute
    513 Broadway
    New York, NY 10012
    (212) 674-7111

Sexuality Information and Education Council of the U.S. (SIECUS)
    130 West 42nd Street, Suite 350
    New York, NY 10036-7802
    (212) 819-9770
    www.siecus.org